Immunohematology and Blood banking

Pritam Singh Ajmani

Immunohematology and Blood banking

Principles and Practice

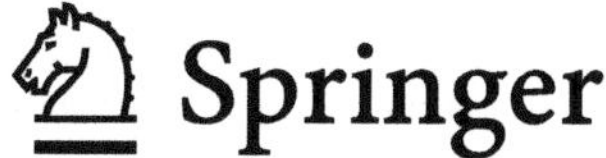

Pritam Singh Ajmani
Ruxmaniben Deepchand Gardi Medical College
Surasa, India

ISBN 978-981-15-8437-4 ISBN 978-981-15-8435-0 (eBook)
https://doi.org/10.1007/978-981-15-8435-0

This Springer imprint is published by the registered company Springer Nature Singapore Pte Ltd.
The registered company address is: 152 Beach Road, #21-01/04 Gateway East, Singapore 189721, Singapore

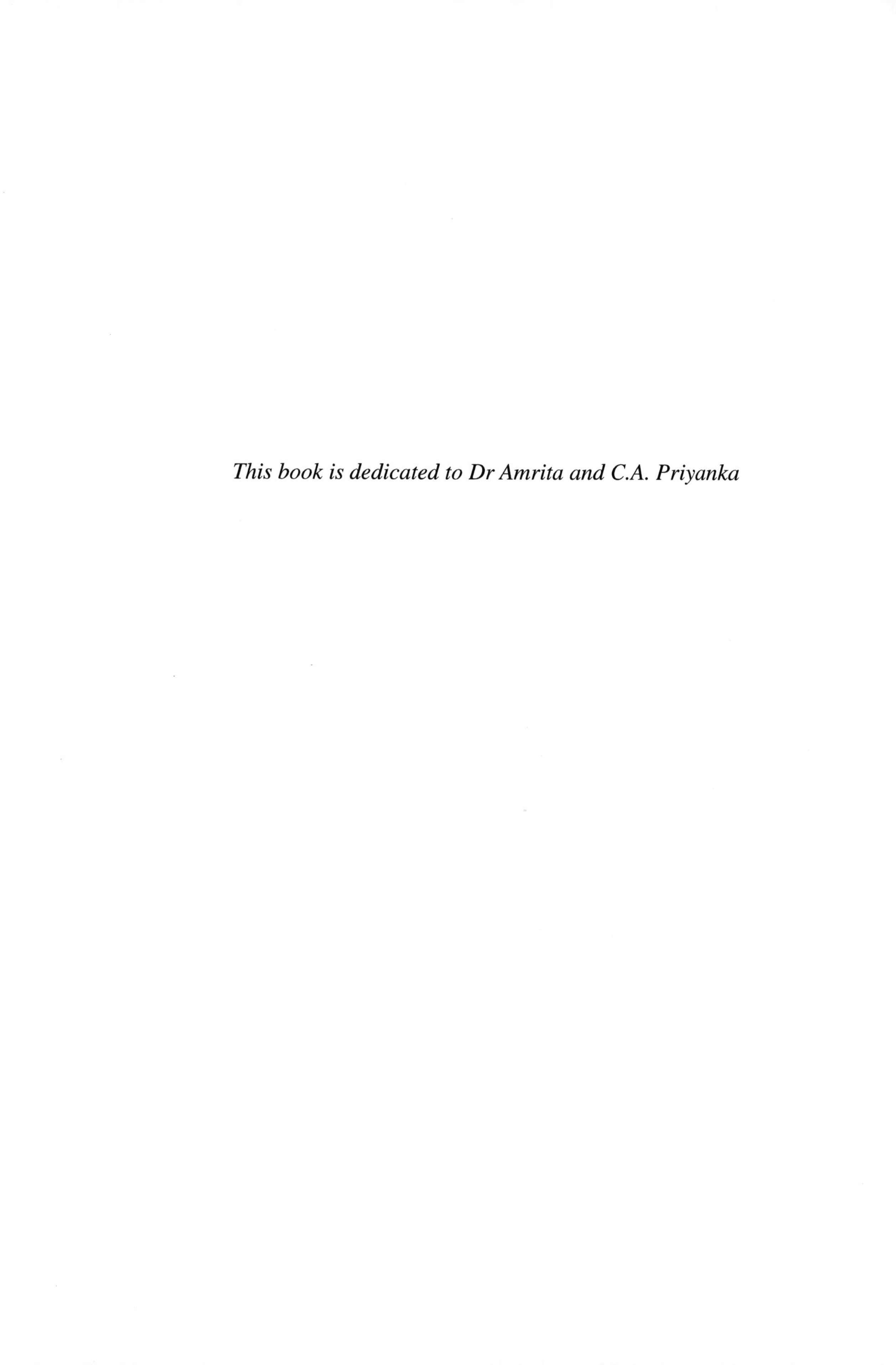

This book is dedicated to Dr Amrita and C.A. Priyanka

Preface

Blood transfusion is one of the most important procedures of modern clinical practice, and over the past two decades blood transfusion science has made tremendous progress. The main aim of blood transfusion is to make transfusion therapy safer. Keeping this thing in mind the need of concise, comprehensive knowledge about transfusion medicine and immunohematology in day-to-day practice, the book has been designed. To achieve this, up-to-date knowledge of evidence-based guidelines for transfusing blood and blood products to benefit the patients is essential. Every day blood transfusions take place routinely and in emergencies to save millions of lives all over the world. To achieve the goal a constant need for regular supply of blood is essential as the shelf life of blood and its components is very less. Regular blood donation by a sufficient number of healthy people is needed to ensure that blood will always be available whenever and wherever it is needed. However, due to resource scarcity, it is not always possible to fulfill the demand of the patient at the right time. Transfusion medicine virtually covers all aspects of immunohematology and laboratory medicine relevant to patient care, health promotion and safer blood transfusion, prevention of transfusion reactions and its management. Appropriate training and knowledge of technological advancement in blood banking is absolutely essential for technical staff for successful implementation of blood banking protocols and timely delivery of blood components to needy patients. Transfusion medicine addresses selection of blood donors, pretransfusion testing, collection of blood, its storage, and separation to different components, indication, and contraindications of blood components therapy.

The book comprises of 15 chapters, each of which begins with specific knowledge of the subject and its practical applications for performance of the test. This book is a navigation guide for undergraduate and postgraduate medical students of all specialty, primary care physicians, pathologists, medical practitioners, paramedical and blood banking personnels. This book is very helpful for medical students and house officers, in the daily practice of pathology, by discussions of various aspects of the subject.

The book is principally designed for global exposure for medical students and faculty members.

The book serves the need of all who has opted postgraduate degree course in pathology and transfusion medicine. It is equally useful for all medical students who are appearing in university examination to prepare their viva voice and for preparation for postgraduate entrance exam with content that is easily assimilated by the reader.

The book is an introductory text designed to provide faculty member in academics with core concept of effective teaching on focused chapters with practicals and labs.

An attempt has been made on a learner-centered perspective and emphasizes outcomes for student learning.

The approach of the book is simple and user friendly. I hope that clinical consultants, pathologists, medical technology students, graduate medical education trainees, resident in pathology and related disciplines will find the book useful. They can use this edition to attain information in the knowledge and learning process, for inpatients care and for continuous reading, to promote continuous medical education and lifelong learning.

Surasa, India P. S. Ajmani

Salient Features of the Book

Comprehensive knowledge of the topics

Update test procedures

Fallacy errors of the test procedures

Interpretation of the test result

Normal reference values

Clinical correlation with disease

Precise preparation of report

Update Literature for Power point presentation & lecture classes for all medical students

Acknowledgements

Writing a medical book about the story of your life is a surreal process. It is harder than I thought and more rewarding than I could have ever imagined. The experience is both internally challenging and rewarding. Any effort becomes successful when there is the effect of synergy—the concept that two and two makes more than four. This book has also the effect of synergy, without prejudice to my own contribution. I wish to start by thanking my daughter Dr Amrita for sharing her truthful and illuminating views on a number of topics related to the book and to my daughter C.A. Priyanka who always cheers me up, never failing in inspiring and encouraging me which helped me to finish this book in half the time. Without their support, it would not have been possible to complete the task.

My deepest and most intimate gratitude is reserved for my awesome wife Rajender for her eternal support and understanding of my goals and aspirations. She is my inspiration and the reason why I work so hard. Her unconditional love and support have always been my strength. Her patience and sacrifice will remain my inspiration throughout my life. It is a boom to me to have such a lovely and caring family, standing beside me with their love and unconditional support. My love for you shall live forever.

I am forever indebted to entire staff of Springer publication for their cooperation tireless, diligent, and meticulous work, careful indexing and editorial help that made getting this book in front of you. Special thanks to, the ever-patient Publishing Manager, and, the greatest cover designer I could ever imagine. I wish to acknowledge the valuable contributions of the reviewers regarding the improvement of quality, coherence, and content presentation of chapters.

I would also like to show my gratitude to Dr Y.K. Mahadik, Medical Director, R.D. Gardi Medical College, Ujjain, for sharing his pearls of wisdom with me during the course of writing this book.

Contents

About the Author

Pritam Singh Ajmani received M.D. Degree in Pathology & Microbiology from Devi Ahilya University, Indore. Presently he is working as Professor of Pathology, in R.D. Gardi medical college, Ujjain. He has 43 year's of experience in teaching & diagnostic pathology. He has served as a consultant pathologist in 350 bedded, Shri Cloth Market Hospital, Indore. The author has done Diploma in Hospital Administration.

1 Introduction

1.1 Introduction

Blood is essential for human life. Blood is an opaque red fluid, freely flowing but denser and more viscous than water. Blood transports oxygen and nutrients to the cells of the body and carries carbon dioxide and other waste products of metabolism. Blood is a tissue and a fluid. It is a tissue because it is a collection of similar specialized cells that serve particular functions. These cells are suspended in a liquid (plasma), which makes the blood a fluid. Plasma is a complex liquid portion of the whole blood containing more than 90% water and contains coagulation factors, antibodies, and various chemicals.

Blood volume is defined as the total amount of blood circulating within the arteries, capillaries, veins, venules, and chambers of the heart at any time. The components that add volume to blood include red blood cells (erythrocytes), white blood cells (leucocytes), phagocytic cells, platelets, and plasma. Plasma comprises about 55% of total blood volume, and erythrocytes make up roughly 45% along with leukocytes and platelets. Normally red blood cells and plasma are fairly uniform in volume. The amount of blood circulating within an individual depends on their age, weight, and size, but the average human adult has nearly 5 liters of circulating blood. Women tend to have a lower blood volume than men. However, a woman's blood volume increases by roughly 50% during pregnancy. A child has more blood volume in relation to his body weight.

The technique of replacing blood and its components is called blood transfusion.

Blood transfusion is a major medical service routinely applied in whole of the world, and it is one of the life-saving interventions. The function of blood bank includes collection of blood from healthy blood donors, storing it at appropriate temperature, processing it, and supplying it to the needy recipients.

The compatibility test is based on the immunological reaction of the red cells of the donor with circulating antibodies present in recipient's plasma under natural conditions.

Compatibility testing is performed to determine ABO and Rh grouping and crossmatching of both donor and recipient to determine the suitability of blood transfusion.

The laboratory testing procedures are based on the visible immunological reaction of hemagglutination and hemolysis.

Definitions of blood product: Any therapeutic medicine or product prepared from human blood

Whole blood: Unseparated whole blood collected into a blood bag containing an anticoagulant as a preservative solution

Blood component is a constituent of blood, separated from the whole blood, such as red cell

P. S. Ajmani, *Immunohematology and Blood banking*, https://doi.org/10.1007/978-981-15-8435-0_1

concentrate, plasma, platelet concentrates, and cryoprecipitate. Plasma or platelets are collected by apheresis. Cryoprecipitate is prepared from fresh frozen plasma.

1.2 Uses of Blood Grouping

For blood transfusion: Before blood donation ABO and Rh (D) grouping is vital for compatible donor. The remaining red cell antigen systems are not of clinical importance in routine blood transfusion.

For organ transplants: The ABO antigens are widely distributed throughout the different body tissues, and for this reason, when organs are transplanted, blood group-specific organ is always chosen.

Paternity test: Blood group studies are not used to prove paternity, but it provides unequivocal evidence that a male is not the father of a particular child. Since the red cell antigens are inherited as dominant traits, a child cannot have a blood group antigen that is not present in one or both parents. For example, if the child in question belongs to group A and both the mother and the father belongs to group O, the man is excluded from paternity. By using multiple red cell antigen systems and additional studies on other blood group types, like MN grouping, red cell enzyme study, human leukocyte antigen (HLA), and plasma proteins provides high degree of statistical certainty that a particular male is the father (Table 1.1).

Table 1.1 Exclusion of paternity on the basis of ABO grouping

Mother and father group	Offspring	Impossible children
A and A	O, A	B, AB
A × B	O, A, B, AB	
A × AB	A, B, AB	O
O × O	O	A, B, AB
O × B	O, B	A, AB
O × A	O, A	B, AB
O × AB	A, B	O, AB
B × B	O, B	A, AB
B × AB	A, B, AB	O
AB × AB	A, B, AB	O

1.2.1 Exclusion of Paternity on the Basis of MN Grouping

The laws of inheritance of MN factors are derived from general principles of Mendelian inheritance. A child cannot possess M or N unless these factors are present in the blood of one or both parents. A parent of type M cannot have a child of type N. A parent of type N cannot have a child of type M. A child of blood type M must have inherited the M factor from both the parents. The same applies to N factor. The MN type has inherited the M factor from one parent either mother or father and the N factor from the other parent either mother or father.

Where blood type of mother and child is known, the father is ruled out as follows (Table 1.2):

Mutations are extremely rare in the MNS; for this reason it is most often applied for paternity test. The test can be performed only at specialized center due to the fact that sufficient quantities of potent and specific antisera are not always available.

The forensic medicine: By inhibition test antigens on red cells can be identified in blood stains on the samples taken from the site of crime in forensic medicine.

Anthropological study of different populations: The blood groups are found in all humans but vary in frequency. An analysis of populations yields striking differences in the frequency of some blood group genes. The O gene is common throughout the world. The maximum frequency of the B gene occurs in northern and central India. The frequency of the A gene is the highest among the Blackfoot Indians of Montana and the Sami people of northern Scandinavia and Australian Aborigines.

Table 1.2 Paternity test on the basis of MN grouping

Mother's blood type	Child's blood type	Father cannot be
N	N	M
MN	M	N
M	M	N
MN	N	M
M	MN	M
N	MN	N

1.3 Discovery of Human Blood Groups

Jan Janský a Czech serologist had independently pioneered the classification of the human blood group. In 1900, Karl Landsteiner, an Austrian biologist and physician, discovered reactions between the RBCs and serum were related to the presence of markers (antigens) on the RBCs and antibodies in the serum. This led to the discovery of ABO blood group and classification of blood groups A, B, and C. He later changed blood group C to O. He was awarded Nobel Prize in Physiology or Medicine in 1930 for his discovery. He was also awarded Albert Lasker Award (referred as America's Nobel Prize) posthumously along with Alexander S. Wiener. He is being considered as the Father of Transfusion Medicine. A fourth blood group AB was discovered by Von Decastello and Sturli in 1902. This testing gave rise to red cells carrying A antigen, cells carrying B antigen, cells carrying both A and B antigens, and cells that do not carry either A or B antigen labeled as group O (implying zero antigen). These blood group antigens were established by reacting with their corresponding antibodies present in the serum of a different blood group. This **immunological reaction is termed as hemagglutination reaction**, which has given the pathway for fundamental concept of blood banking and thus paved the way for blood transfusions to be carried out safely. A person with group B have B antigen on the surface of red cells and A antibody in serum. A person with blood group A have A antigen on red cells and anti-B antibody in the serum. A person with AB blood group has both A and B antigens on the red cells and no anti-A nor anti-B antibody in serum. A person with blood group O (null) has neither A nor B antigens on the surface of RBCs but has both A and B antibodies in blood plasma. For example, people with type B blood will have the B antigen on the surface of their red cells. As a result, anti-B antibodies will not be produced by them because they would cause the destruction of their own blood. However, if A type blood is injected into their systems, anti-A antibodies in their plasma will recognize it as alien, resulting in agglutination of the transfused red cells in order to cleanse the blood of alien protein.

1.3.1 Blood Tests for Transplant

There are three main blood tests to determine if a patient and a potential donor are suitable for a kidney transplant. They are blood typing, tissue typing, and crossmatching.

1.3.2 Blood Typing

Donors with blood type O can donate to recipients with types A, B, AB, and O.

Donors with blood type B can donate to recipients with blood types B and AB.

Donors with blood type A can donate to recipients with blood types A and AB. Donors with blood type AB can donate to recipients with blood type AB only. The Rh factor positive or negative of blood does not matter. The following blood types are compatible:

1.3.3 Selection of Donor for Organ Donation

Recipients with blood type A can receive a kidney from blood types A and O.

Recipients with blood type B can receive a kidney from blood types B and O.

Recipients with blood type AB can receive a kidney from types A, B, AB, and O.

Recipients with blood type O can receive a kidney from blood type O only.

Tissue typing: The best match for the recipient is to have 12 out of 12 antigen matches. (This is known as a zero mismatch.) It is possible for all 12 markers to match, even with an unrelated deceased donor organ, if the patient has a very common HLA type.

Blood test measures antibodies to HLA: This test is done for the patient only and is repeated frequently. HLA antibodies can be harmful to the transplanted organ, and their titer can be increased or decreased over time, so they must be measured while waiting for a transplant, immediately before a transplant surgery, and sometimes following transplantation.

If a patient has HLA antibodies in their blood, they are considered HLA "sensitized," and the donor is not suitable for organ donation. HLA antibody levels can change following events such as blood transfusions, miscarriages, and minor surgeries (including dental work or fistula replacement).

Hemagglutination reaction occurs when an individual is exposed to foreign tissues, either through a blood transfusion, pregnancy, or previous transplant; individual can develop an antibody to different HLA proteins. If a person is positive for HLA antibodies, he is considered "sensitized," and PRA percentage will be greater than 0. The more HLA antibodies in blood, the higher is the PRA percentage. HLA antibody test is indicated immediately before transplant for the HLA antibodies can vary over time; hence the percentage of PRA can also change.

1.3.4 Serum Crossmatch

Serum crossmatch is indicated multiple times, including just before the transplant surgery. To do the test, cells from the donor are mixed with patient's serum. If serum has antibodies against the donor's cells, the antibodies will bind the donor cells and be detected using a fluorescent detection method. If these antibodies are at high levels, the donor cells will be destroyed. This is called a positive crossmatch, and it means that the transplant cannot take place. To do so would result in immediate rejection of the transplanted kidney.

1.3.5 Types of Donor for Organ Transplant

Living related donors (LRD)) are donors who are blood relatives of the recipient.

Living unrelated donors (LURD)) are not blood related and are usually spouses or friends of the recipient.

A third type of living donor is called an altruistic donor or non-directed donor.

Change of blood group: an individual has the same blood group for life, but very rarely an individual's blood type changes through addition or suppression of an antigen in underlying conditions:

Infection: A number of illnesses may alter a person's ABO phenotype. Patients can "acquire" the B antigen during a necrotizing infection during which bacteria release an enzyme into the circulation that converts the A_1 antigen into a B-like antigen. During this time, patients should not receive blood products that contain the B antigen because their sera will still contain anti-B. Once the underlying infection is treated, the patients' blood groups return to normal.

Illness: This can also cause patients to "lose" ABO blood group antigens. Any disease that increases the body's demand for RBCs may weaken the expression of ABO blood group antigens, e.g., **thalassemia.**

Malignancy : Hematological cancers that can modify the sugar chains that bear the ABO blood group antigens, lending to the use of the A and B antigens as tumor markers for acute leukemia, myeloproliferative disorders, and myelodysplasia.

Autoimmune disease: Multiple sclerosis.

Bone marrow transplant: The recipient blood type will eventually change to the donor type. For example, if recipient had a blood type A + prior to transplant and a donor had a blood type of O, eventually recipient blood type would become O. It may take several weeks, and possibly months, for original blood type to disappear, but eventually it will.

Further Reading

Chakraborty RA, Shaw M, Schull WJ. Exclusion of paternity: the current state of the art. Am J Human Genet. 1974;26(4):477.

Dean L. The ABO blood group. In: Blood Groups and Red Cell Antigens [Internet]: National Center for Biotechnology Information (US); 2005.

Garovoy MR. Flow cytometry analysis: a high technology crossmatch technique facilitating transplantation. Transplant Proc. 1983;15:1939–44.

Lee L. Volume of blood in a human. The Physics Factbook; 1998.

Pattinson S. Designing donors. Cardiff Centre for Ethics, Law and Society. Issue of. the Month. 2003;

Table of Blood Group Systems. International Society of Blood Transfusion. October 2008. Archived from https://www.isbtweb.org/fileadmin/user_upload/files-2015/red%20cells/general%20intro%20WP/Table%20blood%20group%20systems%20v4.0%20141125.pdf

World Health Organization. Meeting on WHO Guiding Principles on Human Organ Transplantation, 8–10 June 2009, Kuala Lumpur, Malaysia: report. Manila: WHO Regional Office for the Western Pacific; 2009.

2 Blood Group and Immunology

2.1 Introduction

At the beginning of the twentieth century, an Austrian scientist, Karl Landsteiner, observed in his experiment that the RBCs of some individuals were agglutinated by the serum from other individuals. He observed the patterns of agglutination and showed that blood could be divided into different groups on the basis of agglutination. This marked the discovery of the first blood group system, ABO, and Landsteiner earned a Nobel Prize.

Landsteiner explained that the reactions between the RBCs and serum were due to the presence of markers (antigens) on the RBCs and antibodies in the serum. Agglutination occurred when the RBC antigens were bound by the antibodies in the serum. He called the antigens A and B, and depending upon which antigen the RBC expressed, blood either belonged to blood group A or blood group B. A third blood group contained RBCs that reacted as if they lacked the properties of A and B, and this group was later called "O" after the German word "Ohne," which means "without." The following year, the fourth blood group, AB, was added to the ABO blood group system. These RBCs expressed both A and B antigens.

ABO and Rh (D) group remains the most important in transfusion medicine and transplantation surgery since any person above the age of 6 months possesses clinically significant anti-A and/or anti-B antibodies in their serum.

In 1910, researchers proved that the RBC antigens were inherited and that the A and B antigens were inherited co-dominantly over O. There was initially some doubts over how a person's blood type was determined, but the difficulty was solved in 1924 by Bernstein's "three allele model." The ABO blood group antigens are encoded by one genetic locus, the ABO locus, which has three alternative (allelic) forms—A, B, and O. A child receives one of the three alleles from each parent, giving rise to six possible genotypes and four possible blood types (phenotypes).

Karl Landsteiner discovered that blood clumping was an **immunological reaction** which occurs when the receiver of a blood transfusion has antibodies against the donor blood cells. His work made it possible to determine **blood types** and thus paved the way for blood transfusions to be carried out safely.

Following the discovery of ABO blood group, **Mendelian law of inheritance 1924** of blood groups was well established. After advancement in transfusion therapy, transfusion became more and more common in day-to-day clinical practice, and the detection of immune antibodies became evident. These immune antibodies were developed as a result of incompatible transfusions.

P. S. Ajmani, *Immunohematology and Blood banking*, https://doi.org/10.1007/978-981-15-8435-0_2

The term "blood group" encodes the entire blood group system comprising red blood cell (RBC) antigens whose specificity is controlled by a series of genes which can be allelic or linked very closely on the same chromosome.

"**Blood type"** refers to a specific pattern of reaction to testing antisera within a given system. Upon further advancement understanding on blood group has evolved to encompass not only transfusion-related problems but also specific disease association with RBC surface antigens.

2.2 Principles of Immunohematology

Before going into the details of blood transfusion procedures and reactions, it is important to understand the basic principles in immunohematology and different clinical terms.

Immunology: It deals with the immune system and the cell-mediated and humoral aspects of immunity and immune responses. It is the study of resistance (immunity) to disease. Immunological study comprises all aspects of the immune system, including its structure and function, disorders of the immune system, immunization, blood banking, and organ transplantation.

Immunohematology: A branch of immunology that deals with the immunological properties of the blood. It is the study of antigen–antibody reactions and analogous phenomena as they relate to the pathogenesis and clinical manifestations of blood disorders.

Antigens: Antigens are toxins or foreign substances which when introduced into the body can induce an immune response by the formation of antibodies.

Antigens and their specific antibodies react with each other when they come in contact. Red cell antigens are the blood group factors which reside on the surface of the red cell membrane. They may also be present in various body tissues and fluids. These antigens are mostly proteins and glycoproteins. So more than 410 antigens have been discovered on the surface of red cells. The clinical relevance of these antigens for blood component transfusion and tissue or organ transplantation lies in the ability of these surface molecules to incite an immune response. In addition, some RBC surface antigens have cellular functions with clinical relevance, and others are targets of immune attack in certain infections.

2.2.1 The Basic Blood Group System ABO

The basis for human blood group system is the antigenic characters of red cells.

Human beings could be classified into four groups depending on the presence of one (A) or another (B) or both (AB) or none (O) of the antigens on their red cells.

The presence of antibodies in the plasma follows the Landsteiner's law which states that the corresponding antibody is never present in serum of an individual when the antigen is manifest on his red cells. The antibody against ABO group system are naturally present without any evident antigenic stimulation.

It was later found that A and B are not the only antigens present on the red cells. There are many other antigens, and some of them are capable of producing immune antibodies in the recipient's blood when the latter receives antigen that is foreign in red cell antigen (not present on the red cell of recipient). These immune antibodies will react in subsequent transfusion with the same antigen which proved to be inert during the first transfusion. This observation led to the discovery of other blood group system.

Since the discovery of the ABO system, there are nearly 300 blood group systems. Some of clinical importance is listed below, while others are relatively rare (Box 2.1).

Box 2.1: The ABO Antigens Characteristics

Added to proteins or lipids in red cells
A antigen is N-acetyl-galactosamine (GalNac)
Galactose B antigen is galactose
Substrate molecule is H (fucose)
A and B genes code for transferase enzymes

2.2.2 Red Blood Cell Antigens Can Be Proteins or Sugars

Blood group antigens are either sugars or proteins, and they are attached to various components in the red blood cell membrane.

For example, the antigens of the ABO blood group are sugars. They are produced by a series of reactions in which enzymes catalyze the transfer of sugar units. A person's DNA determines the type of enzymes they have and, therefore, the type of sugar antigens that end up on their red blood cells.

In contrast, the antigens of the Rh blood group are proteins. A person's DNA holds the information for producing the protein antigens. The Rh (D) gene encodes the D antigen, which is a large protein on the red blood cell membrane. Some people have a version of the gene that does not produce D antigen, and therefore the Rh (D) protein is absent from their red blood cells.

The antigenic characters of red cells are inherited. The antigen composition of all blood groups, as determined in the laboratory, is the phenotype, based on the serologic reaction of red cells (hemagglutination) with the corresponding antibody. Thus, AA or AO antigens on the red cells will react equally with anti-A, and the cells will be grouped as A. The genotype, that is the actual genetic character responsible for the phenotype (AA & AO), can only be deduced by tracking the family history of blood type (Box 2.2).

Box 2.2: Diseases Associated with ABO Blood Group Antigen

Blood group	Disease
A	Gastric carcinoma
O	Duodenal ulcer
Absence of Rh antigens	Stomatocytes of Red cells
Duffy negative Red cells	Resistant to *Plasmodium knowlesi*

The ABO blood group antigens are encoded by one genetic locus, the ABO locus, which has three alternative (allelic) forms—A, B, and O. A child receives one of the three alleles from each parent, giving rise to six possible genotypes and four possible blood types (phenotypes).

Table 2.1 Showing genotypes of different blood groups

Blood group	Antigen(s) on RBCs	Antibodies in serum	Genotype
O	A antigen none	Anti-A and Anti-B	OO
B	B antigen	Anti-A	BB or BO
AB	A antigen + B antigen	None	AB
A	A antigen	Anti-B	OO AA or AO

Inheritance of the antigenic character of red cells follows **Mendel's First Law of Inheritance of 1924.** Each antigen is controlled by a gene, which is the unit of inheritance.

The ABO gene locus is located on the chromosome 9.

A and B blood groups are dominant over the O blood group.

The ABO gene is autosomal (the gene is not either sex chromosome).

A and **B** group genes are **co-dominant.**

Each person has **two copies of genes** coding for their ABO blood group (one maternal and one paternal in origin).

Autosomal chromosome: The alleles for blood group are in the same place on chromosome 9. However the genes have a different code giving the different blood group. Individual traits are inherited separately from each other. Each individual will only have two alleles for the same trait. One allele comes from the mother, and the other comes from the father. Homozygous and heterozygous conditions of the red cell antigen are assessed from the genotype. When both the antigens, which are inherited from the mother and the father, are identical examples (AA), it is called homozygous, and when it is different (AO), it is heterozygous (Table 2.1).

A phenotype consists of only those traits or antigens that can be directly typed, whereas a genotype is the sum of all genes a person has inherited within a blood group system.

2.2.3 What Do Co-dominant Genes Mean?

This signifies that if a person inherited one A group gene and one B group gene, their red cells would possess both the A and B blood group antigens.

Table 2.2 Showing genotypes of the offspring

ABO genotype of the off spring		ABO alleles inherited from the mother		
ABO alleles inherited from the father		A	B	O
	A	A	AB	A
	B	AB	B	B
	O	A	B	O

2.2.4 Nomenclature

These alleles were termed A (which produced the A antigen), B (which produced the B antigen), and O (which was "non-functional" and produced no A or B antigen) (Table 2.2).

2.2.5 Antibodies

Antibodies (also known as immunoglobulins) are large Y-shaped proteins. They are produced by circulating lymphocytes and plasma cells following antigenic stimulation. Antibodies combine chemically with substances which the body recognizes as alien, such as bacteria, viruses, and foreign substances in the blood. The antibodies are found in serum or other body fluids and can be demonstrated serologically by reacting with corresponding antigen (immunological reaction).

Antibodies are the main elements in the adaptive immune system. The antibody recognizes a unique part of the foreign target called an antigen. Antibody against red cells can be present naturally in an individual from birth without any known antigenic stimulation. These are called natural antibody (anti-A and anti-B).

Immune antibodies are produced when red cells carrying the corresponding antigen enter into an individual who normally lacks the invading antigen, for example, anti-D and anti-fy.

The immune and natural antibodies differ in physical and chemical characteristics. The natural antibodies are IgM class with large molecular weight (900,000), whereas the incomplete antibodies are of smaller molecular weight (150,000). This may be the reason why the immune antibodies leak through placental barrier. Non-penetration of the natural antibodies from the mother to the fetus protects the latter from incompatible maternal blood..

Table 2.3 Showing antibody characteristics of IgG and IgM types

Antibody characteristics	IgM	IgG
Reaction enhanced—by enzyme-treating cells	Yes	Yes
Reaction enhanced—by lowering temperature	Yes	No
Readily inhibited by soluble A or B antigens	Yes	No
Inactivated by 2—Me or dithiothreitol	Yes	No
Predominant in non-immunized group A and B donors	Yes	No

Antibodies present in plasma are a part of our immune system. Hence, for the identification of the antibody, clotted blood, which yields serum, is required.

Immune antibodies produced by infectious agents do not interfere normally in the blood banking procedures except in case of mycoplasma infection which causes atypical pneumonia and develop cold-reacting antibodies. These cold-reacting antibodies agglutinate the person's own red cells at 4 °C. Many bacteria are also known to affect the red cell antigens.

Most often the antibody reacts specifically with its corresponding antigen that stimulated its production (D antigen with anti-D). Occasionally, however, two antigens have certain chemical groups in common, and an antibody made against one of them will react to some degree with others. This apparent dual specificity is known as cross reactivity (Table 2.3).

Iso antibodies are antibodies produced by an organism in response to a constituent of their own tissues. They are produced in the same species as the antigen source.

Anti-D (anti-Rh) produced by an Rh-negative fetus, after receiving Rh-positive transfusion of Red cells, is an example of isoantibody production.

Heteroantibodies, however, originate in species other than the source of antigen. The antihuman globulin used in antihuman globulin reaction (Coombs reaction) is a heteroantibody. It is made by injection of human globulin into laboratory animals.

Lectins areplant products with antibody-like characteristics. Examples are anti-A_1 and anti-H.

Immunoglobulin G (IgG): it protects against bacterial and viral infection. It is the most abundant type of antibody and is found in all body fluids.

Immunoglobulin M (IgM)) is the **first** antibody to be made by the body to fight a new infection and is found mainly in the blood and lymph fluid.

2.2.6 Recognition of Immunological Reaction in Blood Banking

The antigen–antibody reaction is widely used in immunohematological laboratory. It is a reversible chemical reaction:

$$\text{Antigen} + \text{antibody} \rightleftarrows \text{antigen} - \text{antibody complex}$$

The forces joining the antigen–antibody complex are not strong covalent bonds but weaker bonds, appropriately named “weak interactions.”

The **clumping together of red blood cells called hemagglutination** is one of the most common visible antigen–antibody reactions applied in blood banking for blood grouping and compatibility testing.

The red cell antigen involved in this process is called agglutinogen, and the antibody that reacts against them is called agglutinin. The natural antibodies like anti-A and anti-B will react with corresponding agglutinogens A&B in saline medium, whereas the immune antibodies like anti-D will react only in a protein medium (albumin) with heat treatment at 37 °C. Various agglutinins, however, require different laboratory conditions for the manifestation of agglutination reaction. The recently introduced modified anti-D antibodies react with D antigen at room temperature without protein (bovine albumin)

2.3 Factors Affecting the Antigen–Antibody Reaction

Temperature is one of the important factors affecting antigen–antibody reaction. Cold-reacting antibodies like anti-M react with the corresponding antigen at low temperature of 4 °C, while others react at room temperature, and a few react only at 37 °C. The degree of reaction of cold-reacting antibodies decreases at higher temperature. Some of the other antibodies like anti-Fy will show no visible agglutination reaction under any of the above conditions. They are detected only by the antihuman globulin test.

Hemolysis is another way of manifesting the antigen-antibody reaction whereby the red cells are hemolyzed releasing cellular content. In this case, the specific antibody (hemolysin) needs a complement which is present in the fresh serum. Some of the blood group antibodies are only agglutinins, whereas others may be agglutinins which appear to become hemolysins in response to antigenic stimulation; the latter, however, once again agglutinate with the destruction of the complement. Complement is thermolabile and is destroyed by heating the serum at 56 °C for 30 min. It may also lose its effect if stored at temperature below 4 °C within 4 days.

2.3.1 Effects of Time

Reactants should be incubated for the optimum time for a good antigen–antibody reaction to develop. Too short an incubation time may not form antigen–antibody reaction; on the other hand, prolonged incubation may cause antigen–antibody complexes to dissociate. The best balance should be determined, documented, and followed each time tests are performed.

2.4 Stages of Immunological Reaction

Immunological reactions occur in two stages:

- Instantaneous combination of the antigen and the antibody
- Manifestation of the above reaction which is relatively slow, leading to hemagglutination, hemolysis, precipitation, or other visible reactions

The completion of the first stage of hemagglutination reaction results in the coating of the antibody on the red cells, a phenomenon known as **adsorption.**

Thus some of the immune antibodies may not produce hemagglutination in the saline medium but will be adsorbed on the red cells carrying corresponding antigen. This is called **sensitization.** The sensitized red cells are recognized by their reaction with the antihuman globulin.

2.4.1 Elution

Antibody attached to the red cell antigen can be separated by the elution process. The sensitized red cells when heated to 56 °C or chemically treated, and centrifuged, the supernatant contains the eluted antibody which was formerly attached to the red cell antigen. There are other methods in which ether or acid is used for the identification of antibodies.

Prozone: For visible immunological reaction, it requires proper proportions of antigen and antibody. An excessive amount of antibody may lead to prozone phenomenon. In this, immunological reaction will not be visible until the antibody is sufficiently diluted. Hence during titration, a positive reaction is not seen in undiluted serum but is visible with diluted serum.

2.5 Summary of Antigen–Antibody Reactions

Antigen–antibody reactions occur in two stages; the first is rapid, and the second takes time for the reaction to become demonstrable.

Centrifugation is the most common way to enhance antigen–antibody reactions.

Hemagglutination occurs when IgM antibodies react with their corresponding red cell antigens.

Sensitization occurs when IgG antibodies react with their corresponding red cell antigens.

Sensitization is not an observable reaction, and potentiators may be employed to allow sensitized cells to agglutinate.

Hemolysis is the result of antigen–antibody reactions utilizing the complement cascade all the way to cell membrane attack and rupture.

Neutralization of antibody occurs in the presence of the corresponding antigen in soluble form. An antibody that has been neutralized cannot thereafter react with red cells containing the corresponding antigen.

Precipitation of soluble antigen and antibody is able to take place when the two reactants are present in the correct proportions. Alternatively, immunodiffusion allows for the development of a precipitin line between antigen and antibody, in an appropriate gel medium.

Many factors influence antigen–antibody reactions; these include the number and site of antigenic determinants on cells, the electric repulsion between red cells, the distance between epitopes, the goodness of fit between antibody and antigen, the immunoglobulin class, the concentration of antibody, as well as the effects of temperature, time, pH, and ionic strength of the surrounding test environment.

Proteolytic enzymes are able to reduce zeta potential, causing sensitized cells to agglutinate.

Enzymes may be used in one- or two-stage techniques; it is important to note, however, that some antigens are modified by enzymes and that their corresponding antibodies will therefore not be detectable in an enzyme medium.

The enzymes in laboratory use include ficin, papain, bromelin, and trypsin.

High molecular mass substances such as polyethylene glycol, albumin, and polybrene are also able to affect zeta potential and cause the agglutination of sensitized cells.

Instead of normal ionic strength saline (NISS), **low ionic strength saline (LISS) is commonly used in antibody detection** tests because incubation time is reduced and antibody uptake is increased. Therefore, the sensitivity of antigen–antibody reactions is enhanced.

Complement which is present in plasma or serum is a protein complex that enhances antigen–antibody reactions. When involved in antigen–antibody reactions, it either leads to lysis or complement fixation (binding to cell walls).

In vitro, complement is labile and adversely affected by temperature and time. Its action is also prevented by anticoagulants, which block calcium, an ingredient required in the complement cascade.

Antihuman globulin (AHG) causes the agglutination of sensitized cells by bridging the gap between them. AHG may be monospecific, or broad spectrum, containing antibodies to both IgG and complement.

2.5.1 The Direct Antiglobulin Test Will Detect Red Cell Sensitization In Vivo

The indirect antiglobulin test is used to determine whether an unknown serum or plasma sample contains IgG antibodies or to determine, when using an IgG grouping reagent, whether a red cell sample contains a particular antigen.

Monoclonal antibodies are produced using hybridoma technology. Each monoclonal antibody is produced from an "immortal" single cell line and produces antibody of exactly the same specificity every time. There is therefore no need for comprehensive standardization from batch to batch in the blood bank, as for human polyclonal antibodies (Tables 2.4 and 2.5).

Table 2.4 Showing comparison of ABO and Rh (D) groups

Parameters	ABO group	Rh (D) group
Gene location	Chromosome 9	Chromosome 1
Antigens	A,B, AB	D
Antigen distribution	Red cells, platelets, body fluids, tissue	Red cells only
Antigen development	Weak expression at birth	Fully developed at birth
Dosage effect	No	Present
Antibody nature	Naturally occurring	Immune
Antibody fixation with complement	Yes	No
Optimal reaction temp	Room temperature	37 °C
Forward grouping	Yes	Yes
Reverse grouping	Yes	No
Antisera	IgM	IgG or IgM
Optimal reaction medium	Saline	Antihuman globulin
Enhancer requirement	No	Yes

Table 2.5 Showing blood groups with natural and immune antibodies

Natural	Immune	Natural + immune (both)
ABO	Rh	P
P	Kidd (Jk)	MNSs
MNS	Duffy (fy)	Kidd (Jk)
Lewis (Le)	Kell(K)	Lutheran(Lu)
Lutheran (Lu)		Li

There are wide variations in antigenic character of red cells. The variations are not only to numerous combinations of antigens but also to their degree of dominance. For example A and B are co-dominant to each other, while both A and B are completely dominant over O. This phenomenon leads to a unique blood type of each individual, and it is just impossible to find two persons. The more complex Rh blood group system has 110 possible types. Taking all the systems and type combinations into account, over 500 billion different types of blood group are possible. Fortunately, only the ABO group system (natural) and Rh system (immune) are of importance in transfusion therapy as they cause serious transfusion reactions in recipient.

2.5.2 The Basic Blood Group System ABO

ABO blood group system is the most important of all blood groups because of the natural presence of A and B antibodies in persons from birth who lack corresponding antigen on his red cells. In addition, transfusion of incompatible ABO blood groups leads to serious transfusion reactions in the recipient.

The A and B antigens on the red cells can be detected very early in fetal life by appropriate laboratory procedures. The receptor sites are, however, not fully developed, and hence, the reactions are not strong. Majority of group A infants appear to belong to subgroup A_2 at birth which later become A_1. The A and B antigenic properties are constant throughout life and demonstrable not only on the red cells but also in various tissue cells and body fluids.

2.5.3 ABO Antibodies

Characters of antibodies present in an individual are not inherited. They develop after antigenic stimulation. The presence of natural antibodies in an individual without known antigenic stimulation is a mystery. Naturally occurring antibodies can be formed after exposure to environmental agents that are similar to red cell antigens, such as bacteria, dust, or pollen. Sensitization through previous transfusions, pregnancy, or injections is not necessary. It is generally believed that that these antibodies are as a result of antigenic stimulation from the AB-like substances so widely distributed in nature. They are IgM antibodies, polyvalent, and react with their corresponding antigens at all temperature in a saline medium. The natural antibodies are unable to cross the placenta and protect the fetus from the mother's incompatible antibodies. Examples of naturally occurring antibodies include anti-B, anti-A, anti-C^w, anti-M, and antibodies in the, Ii, Lewis and P systems. Such antibodies may play a major role in resistance to infection.

The blood group antibodies, anti-A and anti-B, are not normally produced by a newborn infant. It may be assumed that antibody detected in cord blood was passively transferred from maternal circulation. The blood group antibodies (anti-A and anti-B) begin to appear in infant at 3–4 months of age. The titer of the natural antibodies increases through adolescence and then gradually decreases with aging. In general anti-A titers are higher than anti-B, and the anti-A titer of group O individual is usually higher than that of a group B person. All other naturally occurring antibodies are considered "unexpected."

2.5.4 Subgroups of ABO Blood Group System

Von Dungern and Ludwik Hirszfeld discovered the A subgroup as A_1 and A_2 and heritability of ABO groups in 1910–1911. The most common subgroups of group A phenotype are A_1 and A_2 These account for over 99% of individuals who are classified as group A.

2.5.4.1 Subgroups of ABO Blood Group System

The procedures used with this reagent are based on the principle of agglutination described by Landsteiner. Normal human red blood cells possessing antigens will clump in the presence of antibody directed toward the antigens. Anti-A1 lectin (Dolichos biflorus) is used for the detection of the A_1 antigen on human red cells.

Anti-A1 Lectin is a purified extract derived from the seeds of *Ulex europaeus*. This reagent contains a phytohemagglutinin which is virtually specific for the H antigen on human red blood cells and in assessing the H secretor status of group "O" individuals. Erythrocytes possessing the A antigen can be subdivided into A_1 and A_2 cells. Group A red blood cells which are agglutinated with anti-A1 lectin are said to be of subgroup **A_1**. Those which are not agglutinated by anti-A1 lectin fall into subgroups weaker than A1, the majority being classified **as A_2 group**

and approximately 80% of the population of blood group A is $\mathbf{A_1}$**,** while the remaining 20% are A_2 or weaker subgroup. This, therefore, divides groups A and AB into the following subgroups: A_1, A_1B, A_2, and A_2B. These weak phenotypes, in majority of the cases, result from the expression of an alternate weak allele present at the ABO loci. Approximately 2% of individuals who are subgroup A_2 have naturally occurring anti-A_1 in their serum. For confirmation of A_1 subgroup reverse serum grouping is performed, the presence of agglutination confirms the diagnosis A_1 subgroup (Table 2.6).

The subgroups are important in blood transfusion. As evident from the above table, anti-A_1 may be present in A $_2$ person, and also weaker subgroups can be identified as group O recipient. If this misdiagnosed group O blood is given to group O recipient, whose serum contains anti-A_1, a transfusion reaction may occur (Table 2.7).

2.5.5 Variants in the ABO Blood Group System

Variations in the ABO blood group system are occasionally seen which defy the general reactions. These are defective blood groups. They are as follows:

- Existence of subgroups, for example, subgroups of A.
- Defective group O with only anti-B and low or no anti-A is occasionally found. This may be due to the very weak or abnormal A antigen present on the red cells. Similarly the presence of only anti-A and low or no anti-B in blood group O individuals also exists.
- A, B, and AB blood group individuals may occasionally develop a weak anti-H, which prevents these recipients from receiving O group blood which normally has H antigen on their red cells

2.5.6 Bombay Blood Group

Bombay blood phenotype was first discovered in Bombay by Dr. Y. M. Bhende in 1952, named for the city in which it was first discovered. It describes individuals whose RBCs lack the H antigen. The phenotype of Bombay group is O, and genotype is hh. It is a rare blood and can be mistaken as O group.

Antibodies in Bombay group are ant-A, anti-B, and anti-H.

2.5.7 Properties of Bombay Blood Group

- Absence of A, B, and H, antigens on red cells
- No agglutination of red cells with anti-A, anti-B, or anti-H lectin.
- Presence of anti-A, anti-B, and anti-AB antibodies in the serum

Table 2.7 Showing antigens and antibodies in ABO blood groups with subgroups

Blood group	Red cell antigen	Antibody in serum
A_1	A_1	Anti-B
A_2	A_2	Anti-A_1 occasionally found
B	B	Anti-B
A_1B	A_1	None
A_2B	A_2	Anti-A_1 occasionally found
O	Neither A nor B	Anti-A, anti-B

Table 2.6 Showing antigen and antibodies in ABO blood group and its frequency in population

Blood group	Antigens	Antibodies	Frequency		
			Indian	White	Black
A	A	Anti-B	20	40	27
B	B	Anti-A	43	11	20
O	Neither A or B	Both anti-A and anti-B	30	45	49
AB	A and B Both	No anti-A nor anti-B	07	04	04

- Presence of potent, anti-H antibodies in the serum
- Can have A and B gene but cannot synthesize A and B antigens
- Can transfer A and B gene to the next generation
- A, B, H non-secretor (no A, B, or H substances present in saliva)
- Presence of A or B enzymes in serum and red cells
- A recessive mode of inheritance
- Red cells of the Bombay group are compatible only with the serum from another Bombay individual. Due to the presence of anti-H, normal blood group O cannot be given to recipient of Bombay group. The individuals with Bombay blood group can be transfused with autologous blood or blood from individuals of Bombay Oh phenotype only.

Bombay blood group methods: Reverse ABO grouping and anti-H lectin test by slide and tube method.

The most common method to detect Bombay blood group is to perform both forward and reverse typing (both of which will show the same results for a Bombay blood type as one would expect for type O), followed by reverse typing with controls type O cells. The patient's serum or plasma will agglutinate all type O cells except his own.

The slide and tube method for detection of Bombay blood group is described in later pages.

2.5.8 Para-Bombay Blood Group

Para-Bombay red blood cell phenotype can be defined in two ways: weak expression of A, B, and antigens on the red cells and weak expression of H antigen and weak anti-H activity, which is demonstrable only at 4 °C or by using routine absorption and elution techniques. Without the use of anti-H lectin or antiserum, the para-Bombay phenotype would have remained unidentified and the patient grouped as O.

Second type of para-Bombay group in which H antigen is present in the secretions, but there is no expression on red cells. Serum contains anti-H antibodies, and the genotype is (H), Se/Se or Se/se, or se/se.

2.5.9 Plant Agglutinins for ABO Blood Group

Some of the plant products especially coral and beans are found to have properties like anti-A, anti-B, and anti-H. These are called lectins. They are used to detect specific red cell antigens; to activate different types of lymphocytes, in order to resolve problems related to polyagglutination; and so on.

Ulex europaues: Lectins extracted from the seeds of Ulex europaues have anti-H properties on human red cells. They are used for the detection of Bombay blood group.

2.5.9.1 Rh Group

The Rh blood group is one of the most complex and immunogenic blood groups known in humans. The genes that control the system are autosomal co-dominant (chromosome 1) polymorphic (more than 1 phenotype). At present, the Rh system comprises 61 antigens; however new antigens continue to be discovered. The Rh antigens are located on the red cell membrane protein. The D antigen is the most immunogenic and important Rh antigen, followed by c and E. Routine Rh typing of donors and patients only test for the presence or absence of the D antigen. The presence of Rh (D) antigen on red cells confers Rh positivity, while people who lack Rh (D) antigen are Rh negative.

From its discovery in 1939 where it was named (in error) after the Rhesus monkey, it has become second in importance only to the ABO blood group in the field of transfusion medicine for the following reasons:

Exposure of Rh-negative individuals to even small amounts of Rh-positive cells, by either transfusion or pregnancy, can result in the production of Rh antibodies mainly of (IgG) type, in majority of the cases in first instance only.

Secondly hemolytic disease of the newborn occurs as a result of Rh incompatibility of the Rh-negative mother and Rh-positive fetus.

All Rh alloantibodies should be considered potentially capable of causing severe hemolytic transfusion reactions (anti-D, anti-C, anti-e, and anti-c).

Anti-D and anti-c produce severe hemolytic disease of the fetus and newborn. Anti-C, anti-E, and anti-e produce mild to moderate hemolytic disease of the fetus and newborn.

Unlike anti-A and anti-B, which occur as natural antibodies, anti-Rh (anti-D) does not develop without an immunization stimulus. The Rh antigen, like any other red cell antigen, is inherited, but anti-Rh develops in an Rh-negative individual only after the latter receives Rh-positive red cells, or an individual blood circulation is mixed with Rh-positive red cells by any trauma or similar conditions. Stimulus in pregnant female may be any vaginal instrumentation, abortion, miscarriage, and stillbirth. The antigens of the Rh blood group are proteins. A person's DNA holds the information for producing the protein antigens. The Rh (D) gene encodes the D antigen, which is a large protein on the red blood cell membrane. Some people have a version of the gene that does not produce D antigen, and therefore the Rh (D) protein is absent from their red blood cells. To date, 110 Rh antigens are known.

2.5.10 Nomenclature

Number of Rh antigens: 61

ISBT symbol: Rh

ISBT number: 004

Gene symbols: RHD and RHCE

Gene names: Rhesus blood group, D antigen; and, Rhesus blood group, Cc, Ee antigens. The D antigen contains over 30 epitopes.

Incidence of Rh-Negative Varies in Different Races

Antigen Specificity Protein The sequence of amino acids determines the specificity of most of the Rh antigens.

Number of antigens: 61 D, C, E, c, and e are among the most important.

The common alleles are:

C & c are alleles with C^w occasionally seen as a weaker expression of C.

E & e are alleles although E is seen only as third as often e. The e antigen is referred to as a high incidence antigen since it is found in 98% of the population.

D & the lack of D (or d) are alleles.

History of the Rh blood group system was first described in the year 1940.The first case was reported by immunohematologist Philip Levine and physician Rufus Stetson who published their case in *The Journal of the American Medical Association*. They presented an anonymous 25-year-old woman who checked into a local hospital during her 33 weeks of pregnancy complaining of labor pains and vaginal bleeding. The next morning, she delivered an emaciated stillborn fetus weighing only one pound and five ounces. The physicians had to expel the woman's placenta to stop her from bleeding to death. The patient received a blood transfusion from her husband. The recipient had a severe transfusion reaction during the transfusion. Her serum agglutinated red blood cells (RBCs). The following year, Landsteiner and Wiener transfused the red cells of a Rhesus monkey (Rh) into a rabbit. The rabbit produced antibodies (anti-Rh) that were capable of agglutinating the red cells from Rhesus monkeys and also the red cells of 85% of the human population, the remaining 15% of the population red cells did not react with rabbit anti sera were. Those who reacted said to have the Rhesus factor and were Rhesus positive, while those that did not react lacked the Rhesus factor and were Rhesus negative. The terms Rhesus positive, or Rh positive, and Rhesus negative, or Rh negative, are still used (incorrectly) today, especially by clinical doctors and paramedicals to describe what we now know as Rh D positive and Rh D negative. The heteroantibody was renamed anti-LW (after Landsteiner and Wiener), and the human alloantibody was renamed anti-D. By 1945, the original Rh factor had been renamed D and four more antigens were discovered. These were Cc & Ee.

Antihuman serum (Coombs antisera) is used in determining the presence or absence of red blood cell antibody or components of human complement on red blood cells. Accordingly antihuman serum is used for compatibility testing, antibody detection, antibody identification, testing for the variant of the Rho (D) antigen (DU tests), and umbilical cord red blood cell testing.

Bovine albumin is primarily used to enhance the reactivity of blood grouping antibodies, either in direct agglutination tests or indirect antiglobulin test which can be qualitatively used in antibody detection, identification, titration, and control of Rh typing.

2.5.11 Rh Antigen

Rh blood group is a highly complex system with more than 110 antigens identified, but in routine blood bank practice, only 5 basic antigens are of importance.

The different nomenclature is used for Rh-associated antigens. The three most practical nomenclatures are Fisher-Race, Wiener, and Rosenfield (Table 2.8).

Wiener theory: in Wiener theory, agglutinogen means **haplotype,** and factors mean **antigen.** Two genetic systems were originally proposed to explain the relationships and inheritance of these five original Rh antigens. In the USA, Wiener proposed a system in which nomenclature was expressed by the use of a single letter. It is good for describing phenotypes but rarely used. There is one Rh locus which occupies one Rh gene, but this gene has multiple alleles. **Example:** Rh (D), Rh (C), Rh (E), Rh (c), and Rh (e) the gene (d) is an amorphous and has no antigenic expression. So there are only five effective antigens.

Genes are designated by single italic letters R for genes that include Rho(D) and r genes that do not determine Rho, with various superscripts symbols (R^{o} R^{1} R^{2} R^{z} r r′ r^{y} to denotes different alleles). **Gene product (haplotype) designated by Roman type Rh** indicates different haplotype Capital letter R used when the gene product included Rho (D) antigens were indicated by roman character in boldface type ,means Rho represent D & rh′ rh″ hr′ hr″ represent C, E, c, e respectively. Shorthand phenotype notations employ single letter R & r in roman type with subscripts, or superscripts, to indicate antigenic combination. Thus R1 indicates C, D, and e together, and R2 indicates c, D, and e.

Table 2.8 Showing nomenclature of Rh-associated antigens

Fisher–race	Wiener (historical)	Rosenfield
D	Rho	Rh1
C	rh′	Rh2
E	rh″	Rh3
C	hr′	Rh4
E	hr″	Rh 5

2.5.12 Fisher and Race

This system simply describes the presence or absence of the antigen on the RBC. There is no genetic basis. D = 1, C = 2, E = 3, c = 4, e = 5. For example, R1r (DCe/dce): Rh 1, 2, −3, 4, 5 E is number 3; E antigen is not present and is therefore designated with −3

Fisher–Race Example: DCe/DCe individual is homozygous for D, C, and e genes DCe/dcE individual is heterozygous for D, C, e, d, c, and E genes

In the UK, Fisher and Race proposed a system of three closely linked loci for D/d, C/c and E/ each gene coding for the production of a single antigen. Thus, the antigens C and c were thought to be the products of the co-dominant alleles C and c. Antigens E and e were thought to be the products of the co-dominant alleles E and e. The D antigen was the product of the D gene and the proposed allelic gene d was considered an amorphous as no d antigen or anti-d antibody was ever discovered. Fisher also postulated that the order of the genes on a chromosome was DCE. It has become common practice to refer to them in this order. This nomenclature is easy to follow and is currently adopted in most of the laboratories. In the Fisher–Race theory the D gene codes for the D antigen, the C gene codes for the C antigen, etc.

Fisher's system is most complete system and allowed the deduction of phenotypes of offspring from different mating types. Fisher's shorthand notation is very convenient for communicating information regarding phenotypes and genotypes (Table 2.9).

Table 2.9 Showing Rh genotype and its percentage distribution

Rh-positive genotype	Percentage distribution (%)
ccDe	34.7
CCDe	19.03
CcDEe	13.02
ccDEe	11.05
Others	21.03

Table 2.10 Showing Fisher–Race and Wiener nomenclature

Fisher–Race	Antigens	Weiner gene
cDe	D, c, e	R^0
CDe	D, C, e	R^1
cDE	D, c, E	R^2
CDE	D, C, E	R^z
Cde	C, e	*R*
CDe	C, e	r′
cdE	C, E	r″
CdE	C, E	r^y

2.5.13 Difference Between Wiener Theories and Fisher–Race

Wiener theory has only one gene locus at which multiple alleles occur. Fisher–Race theory has three closely linked loci (Table 2.10).

Rosenfield is a numerical system for describing the Rh antigens. This system was free from the genetic implications of either Wiener's or Fisher's systems, as it merely recorded the observed serological reactions. The known Rh antigens were numbered from 1 (for D) to 24, in order of discovery. The numbering of Rh antigens has now reached 110, although, because of obsolete forms, there are now 45 antigens in the system. **The updated system of Rosenfield** refers these antigens as Rh1, Rh2, Rh3, Rh4, and Rh5. Example D+, C+, E−, c+, e+ is written as Rh 1, 2, −3, 4, 5.

The Rh blood group system is controlled by five co-dominant closely linked allelic genes that go together in three pairs Cc, D, and Ee. Presence of "D" antigen cannot be proved because anti-d has not yet been discovered. Thus the absence of "D" antigen is considered as equivalent to the presence of "D" antigen on the red cells. Individuals whose red cells possess "D" antigen, irrespective of the presence or absence of other Rh antigens, are designated as Rh positive. Persons whose red cells lack "D" or Rho are labeled as Rh negative. The other four major antigens are C, E, c, and e; though present in every individual, in some combination, they do not frequently produce strong reacting antibodies. Since every individual has two chromosomes, contributed by the two persons, everyone has two Rh alleles or to decide Rh-related red cell antigen. They may be either identical or different—CDE/CDE or CDE/cde. Fisher–Race states that three pairs of closely linked allelic genes give rise to eight possible antigen combination. At Rh locus, Fisher–Race uses DCE as the order others alphabetize.

DCe	dCe	DcE	dCE	Dce	dcE	DCE	Dce

Fisher–Race Example: DCe/DCe individual is homozygous for D, C, and e genes, and DCe/dcE individual is heterozygous for D, C, e, d, c, and E gene.

Inheritance of Rh group is independent of the ABO group. Approximately 95% of the Indian population is Rh positive and 5% Rh negative. Of the Rh negative, the frequency of cde is higher, while other types Cde, cdE, and CdE are rare.

The presence of all the above-mentioned Rh (C, c, D, E, and e) can be demonstrated by hemagglutination reaction of red cells (Table 2.11).

Table 2.11 Showing identification of Rh antigens by hemagglutination reaction of red cells with knwn antibodies

	Hemagglutination reaction		
Known reagent antibodies	Specimen no 1	Specimen no 2	Specimen no 3
Anti-C	+	+	–
Anti-c	+	–	+
Anti-D	+	+	–
Anti-E	–	–	–
Anti-e	+	+	+
Antigenic character	CcDe	Cde	Cde[a]

[a]Anti-d does not exists and the presence of "d" is indicated by the absence of "D"

2.5.14 Translating from Weiner to Fisher–Race

R refers to D whether it is R^0R1, R2, or Rz.

r refers to the lack of D.

0 refers to having no C or E.

1 or 'refers to C.

2 or '' refers to E.

The very rare haplotypes that have both a C and E are given letters z and y.

Or any time the Rh control is positive, repeat the result.

2.5.15 Rh Antibodies

These antibodies are stimulated following exposure to foreign antigens via transfusion or pregnancy, are IgG in nature of low molecular weight (170,000) than the natural IgM antibody (molecular weight 1,000,000), and do not fix complement. As IgG antibodies, they react best at 37 °C or following antiglobulin testing. They have the capability of causing transfusion adverse events (transfusion reaction, extravascular hemolysis) and, once documented, must continue to be recognized despite a drop in titer below detectable levels. As IgG molecules can cross the placenta, these antibodies must be followed during pregnancy using antibody titration procedures in order to provide useful, timely information regarding its potential to cause hemolytic disease of the fetus and newborn (HDFN). They bind to RBCs and mark them up for destruction in the spleen (extravascular hemolysis). Anti-D, anti-C, anti-e, and anti-c can cause severe hemolytic transfusion reactions. Hemolysis is typically extravascular anti-C, anti-E, and anti-e can cause mild to moderate disease.

Since Rh antibodies are IgG, they bind best at 37 °C, and their reactions will be observed with indirect antiglobulin technique. Agglutination reactions are enhanced by bovine albumin, low ionic strength saline (LISS), proteolytic enzymes (ficin), and polytheylene (PEG).

2.5.16 Dosage Effect

Rh antibodies will react more strongly with homozygous cells than with heterozygous cells. For example, an anti-E will react strongly with E+E+cells and more weakly with E+e+cells. This is called dosage.

Example of dosage: Anti-E may exhibit a 3 + reaction with cells that are E+e– and a 2+ reaction with cells that are E+e+.

2.5.17 Rh Blood Group and Rh Incompatibility

A person with Rh—blood does not have Rh antibodies naturally in the blood plasma (Table 2.12).

2.5.18 Variations of the D Phenotype

They are partial D and weak D. The D antigen contains over 30 epitopes. Variations of the D phenotype arise when these epitopes are only weakly expressed ("weak D phenotype") or when some are missing ("partial D phenotype").

Partial D: In partial D, some D antigen epitopes are missing. The number of D antigens is not reduced, but the protein structure is altered, but in practice, people with partial D are difficult to identify. Individuals whose RBCs carry a partial D phenotype (qualitative D variant with or without weakening of the D antigen) can make alloanti-D. These individuals if alloimmunized to D can produce an anti-D antibody. As a result, they should be considered Rh negative. Therefore, partial D patients who are donating blood should be labeled as D-positive, but, if receiving blood, they should be labeled as D-negative and trans-

Table 2.12 Showing Rh +ve & Rh –ve genotype

Blood type	Genotype	Alleles produced
Rh positive	RR Rr	R R or r
Rh negative	Rr	R

fused with Rh-negative red cells. This phenotype is usually caused by the creation of a hybrid Rh (D) and RhCE protein. The hybrid protein is similar enough to Rh (D) to be correctly inserted in the RBC membrane, but it lacks several epitopes found on the complete Rh (D) protein. Individuals who have been identified as having the "partial D" phenotype should not receive Rh D-positive blood. If a person with the partial D phenotype encounters the complete D antigen on transfused RBCs, they may form anti-D and suffer from a transfusion reaction.

Weak D: In this all D antigen epitopes are present but are underexpressed. This was previously referred to as D^u, which has been replaced by weak D phenotype. Individuals whose RBCs have a weak D phenotype (quantitative D variant) do not make anti-D. "Weak D" is an Rh phenotype found in <1%. It is typically caused by a single amino acid switch in the transmembrane region of the Rh d protein. This disrupts how the Rh d protein is inserted into the RBC membrane, reducing the level of expression of Rhd. In most cases, adequate levels of D antigen are present and because there has been no change in D epitopes, the formation of anti-D is prevented. Therefore, individuals with the weak D phenotype can receive Rh D-positive blood without any adverse effects. Weak D phenotype is characterized by negative reaction with anti-D reagent at immediate spin (IS), negative reaction after 37 °C incubation, and positive reaction at antihuman globulin (AHG) phase. Clinically, weak D individuals of types 1, 2, 3, 4.0, 4.1, and 5 can be treated as Rh positive and be transfused with Rh-positive red cells, while patients with weak type 4.2–11 and 15 should be treated as Rh negative and transfused with Rh-negative red cells (Table 2.13).

2.5.19 Other Blood Group Systems

In addition to ABO and Rh group systems, there are however many other blood group systems which exists side by side, and only the more commonly blood groups will be of importance and discussion. These include Lewis(Le), P, MNS, Kell (K), Duffy(Fy), Kidd (JK), Lutheran(Lu), and Li. These are not routinely done in daily blood bank practice. They are also of clinically significant because the antibodies to some of these blood groups can be naturally present (anti-P), while others will develop following incompatible transfusion(anti-K). Some of them are also implicated in hemolytic disease of the newborn. In order to understand the behavior of other blood group systems, some of the basic rules of ABO and Rh systems may be repeated at this point as they will be applicable here too. All antigenic characters are inherited.

The antibodies may be present from birth (natural like anti-A, anti-B), or they may develop following immunization (immune antibodies, like anti-D)

The specific antibody (natural or immune) will be found only in an individual who lacks the corresponding antigen.

There are 34 other blood group systems with more than 300 known variants. These are all classified by the "antigens" found on the surface of red blood cells. Antigens are molecules (most often proteins, but also carbohydrates) capable of provoking our immune systems to attack.

Blood group "S/s variants" is named after Sydney, where the blood group was discovered. This blood group is signified by a particular type of molecule on the red blood cells that is a target of the malaria parasite.

Table 2.13 Showing laboratory diagnosis of Weak D & partial D

Immediate spin		37 °C anti D		AGT		
Anti-D	Rh (C)[a]	Anti-D	Rh(C)[a]	Anti-D	Rh(C)[a]	Interpretation
+	0					D Positive
0	0	0	0	+	0	Weak D
0	0	0	0	0	0	D negative
0	0	0	0	+	+	

[a]C stands for control

2.5.20 Blood Groups with Natural and Immune Antibodies

Blood groups include Lewis (Le), P, MNS, Kell (k), Duffy (Fy), Kidd (JK), and Lutheran (Lu). These blood groups are not routinely determined in blood bank except in investigation of transfusion reaction. Antibodies to some of these blood groups are naturally present (anti-P), while others will develop following incompatible transfusion (anti K).

2.5.21 MNS and P Blood Group

There are two types of antibodies found in MNS and P groups. They are both natural and immune antibodies. **Natural antibodies** of MNS and P group are cold reactive and react best at a temperature of 4 °C. They seldom cause transfusion reactions because the immunological reaction at the body temperature of 37 °C. **The immune antibodies** of MNS & P group react at 37 °C which is enhanced by the presence of albumin. These immune antibodies are detected by antihuman globulin (Coombs) test.

The presence of MN antigens on red cells is recognized from birth. There is an equal distribution of positive and negative MN traits. MN genotype test is very useful in paternity test of the disputed child.

Lutheran Blood Group: Anti-Le is hemolytic antibody and patient's with anti-Le^a should be given Le (a-). This does not create major problem since four out of five donors are Le (a-) anti-Le antibody reacts over a wide range of temperature and may hemolyze red cells. Le-positive individuals are secretors, and they secrete water-soluble antigens into the body fluids which can be detected in saliva.

Lutheran (Lu) blood group has some unique features. There are two types of antigens on red cells; they are "I" and "i." In the fetal life "i" is the predominant antigen and is readily detected; hence at the time of birth, cord red cells react strongly with anti i. Gradually "I" antigen replaces "i" antigen and at a later stage of life. After 2 years, the red cells react strongly with anti-I antiserum but weakly with anti i. Anti-I antibody is autoantibody and develops without any external stimulation. It may lead to cold reactive autoimmune hemolytic anemia. Anti-I can agglutinate its own red cells at 4 °C (cold agglutinins) and may cause diagnostic problems in crossmatching due to high titer with persistent agglutinating activity even at 37 °C.

Antibodies can be natural or immune. The immune antibody will be found in persons who lack the corresponding antigen and receive blood transfusion the reactive antigen.

2.5.22 Miscellaneous Blood Groups (Human Leukocyte Antigen)

2.5.22.1 HLA

The HLA loci are part of the genetic region known as major histocompatibility complex. HLA is extremely polymorphic which give rise to the production of unique antigenic specificity that is expressed on cell surface and that can be detected by specific antibodies or immunologically activated T cells. Currently, a match between the human leukocyte antigen (HLA) in the sera of the donor and the recipient is the best pre-transplant biomarker. HLA proteins are found in the membranes of nearly every cell in the body in (all cells that have nucleus). These antigens are especially high in concentration on the surface of leukocytes. HLA antigens are present on leukocytes, platelets, and tissue cells. Because the HLA antigens occur on all nucleated cells of the body, they are therefore most important in the body's immune system in transplant survival. Compatibility of HLA antigen between the donor and recipient is necessary in cases of organ transplant (Table 2.14).

Table 2.14 Showing blood group compatibility in blood transfusion

Blood group of donor				
Recipient group	Group A	Group B	Group AB	Group O
A	Yes	No	No	Yes
B	No	Yes	No	Yes
AB	Yes	Yes	Yes	Yes
O	No	No	No	Yes

2.5.22.2 Universal Recipient

People with type AB blood are considered universal recipient, and they can receive blood from a person with any blood type. Their blood does not contain either anti-A or anti-B natural antibodies against the ABO blood groups, and this avoids incompatibility reactions.

2.5.22.3 Universal Donor

Persons belonging to type O blood are considered the universal donor, and their blood can be given to individuals of any other blood group. The red cells of group O do not carry either A or B antigens, and hence they do not react with their corresponding antibodies

The universal plasma donor has type AB blood.

The universal plasma recipient is O positive.

Rare blood group: A person is considered with rare blood group if he lacks antigens that 99% of the people are positive for.

Extremely rare blood group: A person is considered with extremely rare blood group if he lacks antigens that 99.99% of the people are positive for.

2.5.22.4 Rh_{null} Disease

It was first discovered in an Aboriginal Australian and is extremely rare, with fewer than 50 individuals known to have Rh_{null} blood in the 50 years after its discovery.

2.5.22.5 Characteristics

- Absence of all Rh antigens on RBCs
- Short life span of RBC
- Increased osmotic fragility
- Increased Hb –F
- Mild or moderate chronic hemolytic anemia
- Characteristics stomatocytosis on peripheral blood smear examination (Table 2.15)

Table 2.15 Showing antigens and antibodies in ABO group

Blood group	Antigen A	Antigen B	Antibody anti-A	Antibody anti-B
A	Yes	No	No	Yes
B	No	Yes	Yes	No
O	No	No	Yes	Yes
AB	Yes	Yes	No	No

Further Reading

Avent ND, Reid ME. The Rh blood group system: a review. Blood J Am Soc Hematol. 2000;95(2):375–87.

Concept 1: Reviewing Mendel's Laws. The Biology Place. Pearson High School. Archived from http://www.phschool.com/science/biology_place/biocoach/inheritance/laws.html

Daniels G. Human blood groups. 2nd ed. Cambridge, MA: Blackwell Science; 2002.

Daniels G, Poole J, De Silva M, Callaghan T, MacLennan S, Smith N. The clinical significance of blood group antibodies. Transf Med. 2002;12(5):287–95.

Dean The ABO blood group "... A number of illnesses may alter a person's ABO phenotype ...'; 2005.

Letsky EA, Leck IN, Bowman SK. Rhesus and other haemolytic diseases. In: Antenatal & neonatal screening; 2000.

Reid ME, Lomas-Francis C, Olsson ML. The blood group antigen factsbook: Academic Press; 2012.

Scott ML. ES05. 01 The complexities of the Rh system. Vox sanguinis. 2004;87:58–62.

Universal Acceptor and Donor Groups. Webmd.com. 2008-06-12. Archived from https://www.webmd.com/a-to-z-guides/blood-types-what-to-know#2

Wiener AS. Genetics and nomenclature of the Rh-Hr blood types. Antonie van Leeuwenhoek. 1949;15(1):17–28.

Yamamoto F. ABO blood group system—ABH oligosaccharide antigens, anti-A and anti-B, A and B glycosyltransferases, and ABO genes. Immunohematology. 2004;20(1):3.

Your Blood—A Textbook About Blood and Blood Donation (PDF). Archived from the original (PDF) on June 26, 2008, p. 63. Archived from http://www.hartcountyga.gov/documents/Anatomy1blood.pdf

3 Donor Blood Collection

3.1 Blood Collection

Collection of whole blood is one of the most important functions of blood bank. Information collected from the donor and subsequent blood collection is essential prerequisites for successful collection.

3.1.1 Essential Issues in Consent

Voluntary nature of the procedure

Importance of answering questions truthfully

Information about the use[s] of their donation

Ownership of the donation: Data protection aspects and traceability, donor cannot ask the information to be removed from database.

Donor rights: Donor cannot be insisted for donation, but must be explained in details that the donation is not harmful and motivated with courtesy.

3.2 Donor Screening Ethical Issue

- What information should be provided to donor?
- Different methods to ask personal questions?
- Attitude during the interview
- Data security
- High-risk group donors
- Screening test results
- Information to the spouse
- Information to the employer
- Information to the recipients
- Treatment of the recipients
- Recalling of all blood product

3.2.1 Donor Signature

The donor must sign the donor questionnaire in the presence of attending doctor and countersigned by doctor for obtaining the health history confirming that the donor has:

Read and understood the literature provided

Given the opportunity to ask questions

Had been provided with satisfactory responses to any questions asked

Given informed consent to proceed with the donation process

3.3 Donor Interview

Purpose: To insure the quality of blood drawn and to make sure that the loss of donated blood will not harmful for the donor. It includes relevant factors that may help in identifying and screening out persons whose donation could present a health risk to others, such as the

P. S. Ajmani, *Immunohematology and Blood banking*, https://doi.org/10.1007/978-981-15-8435-0_3

possibility of transmitting diseases, or health risks to themselves.

All information provided to donors will be treated in the strictest confidence.

Provide the health and lifestyle questionnaire to read and complete the quest.

Take a donor interview to determine if he is eligible to donate or not.

If donor is not eligible, explain to him in full confidence the reasons for not taking the blood.

3.3.1 Essentials Criteria for Blood Donors

The following are some of the important criteria universally accepted for donor selection:

Unpaid volunteers, donating regularly, are key persons for safe blood donation.

18- to 70-year-olds can enroll as first-time blood donors, and there is no upper age limit for regular donors subject to free from any medical illness.

World Blood Donor Day: June 14 (Box 3.1)

Box 3.1: Showing Essential Criteria for Donor to Donate Blood

Hemoglobin male: 12.5, PCV > 41
Female Hb > 12.5 & PCV > 38
Pulse 60–100 regular
Blood pressure: Systole >120 mmHg
Diastole: >80 mmHg
Temperature: Normal 37.5 °C
Interval between donations: More than 16 weeks
Donor weight >50 kg
Absence of any chronic disease

3.3.2 Predonation Evaluation of Donor

Medical history and risk factor assessment

Testing blood for infectious diseases

The following tests are indicated from the donor blood before donation, and if found normal, donors can donate the blood. Test can also be performed after donation of blood from the blood collected in pilot tube. Blood donor with high-risk category should be first subjected for blood test for infectious diseases, and if found normal, then blood donation should be performed.

ABO and Rh typing

Hepatitis B antigen testing

Hepatitis C antibody testing

HIV 1 and HIV 2 antibodies testing

HTLV 1 and 2 antibodies

Serologic test for syphilis

CMV antibody for selected donor

Hemoglobin determination by copper sulfate method: this method is based on the relationship of specific gravity to hemoglobin concentration. It is used to check that a donor has normal hemoglobin level to be eligible to give blood. Two strengths of $CuSO_4$ solution are normally used, each of which has a different specific gravity: one for male donor with a specific gravity of 1.055 (equivalent to 13.5 g/dL of hemoglobin) and one for female donors with a specific gravity of 1.053 (equivalent to 12.5 g/dL of hemoglobin). In this method, a drop of blood is allowed to fell gently at a height of about 1 cm above the surface of the $CuSO_4$ solution. If the drop of blood has a satisfactory hemoglobin concentration, it will sink in the solution within 15 s. A sample with decreased hemoglobin level will either remain suspended or will sink slightly and then rise to the top of the solution within 15 s.

3.3.3 Guidelines Before Taking the Blood from Donor

Drinking sufficient amount of water in the 24 h prior to donation and eating salty snacks the night before donation will greatly reduce the risk of fainting during or after donation of blood. Advice donor to eat something 4 h prior to blood donation.

Although a donation only takes approximately 20 min, donor has to stay in blood bank for 3 h for the entire process, i.e., from the time for registration to refreshments after the donation. The time taken for different steps is as under:

Donor questionaries' and consent process: 30 min

Investigation on donor blood: 2 h

Donation process: 15 min

Post donation care: 15 min

Total period: 3 h

In case blood investigations on donor blood after collection of donated blood, it will take 2 h.

3.3.4 Donor Session Records Registration and Donor Identification

Donors must positively identify themselves by volunteering their name, date of birth, and permanent address by Aadhar card, voter card, or any of the documents. The identity of the donor must be recorded and linked to the donation record. Once registered, for subsequent identification, their name and date of birth is sufficient.

In case of deferred donors, record the full details and action taken.

3.3.5 Formula for Blood to Be Drawn

Volume of blood to be drawn is determined by the following:

$$\frac{\text{Donor weight in kg} \times 450\,\text{mL}}{55}$$

Example: If whole blood is to be drawn from a donor who weight 50 kg, the calculation would be:

$$50/55 \times 450 = 392\,\text{mL of blood to be drawn}$$

3.4 Blood Donor Questionaries' Form

Date

Confidential

Please answer the following questions correctly. This will help to protect you and the patient who receives your blood.

Full name

First name Last name

Male/Female

Birth date

Age

Father's full name

Father's first name Father's last name

Occupation: organization

Telephone number with area code

Mobile number

Would you like us to call you on your mobile: Yes/No?

Would you like your name to include in donor's website?

E-mail address of donor

Have you donated previously?: Yes/No
If yes, how many occasions
When last: month/date/year
Did you have any discomfort during or after in the previous donation? Yes? No
Your blood group
Time of last meal HH: MIN: AM/PM
Do you feel well today? Yes/No
Did you sleep well last night? Yes/No

Medical Questionnarie
The following questions are included in medical history:

- Do you suffer recently from?
- Corona virus infection
- Flu
- Sore throat
- Fever
- Infection: if positive deferred till donor is recovered.
- In the past 5 months, have you had any history of the following?
- Unexplained weight loss
- Repeated uncontrolled diarrhea
- Swollen salivary glands
- Generalized lymphadenopathy
- Continuous low-grade fever
- Fainting spells
- Dental extraction recent and old within 6 months
- Do you have diabetes?
- In the past 5 months, have you consulted a doctor for a health problem, had surgery, or medical treatment?
- In the past 5 months, have you had Hepatitis? B and C
- In the past 5 months, have you received blood or blood products?
- In the past 12 months, have you had a graft?
- In the past 12 months, have you had close contact with a person who has had hepatitis or jaundice?
- Since 1980, did you receive a blood transfusion or blood products?
- Have you ever had malaria?
- Have you ever had a positive test for the HIV/AIDS virus?

Table 3.1 Showing history of drug essential for donor

Anti-arrhythmic drugs	Immunosuppressive
Anticonvulsants	Growth hormone
Anticoagulants	Sedative
Antithyroid drugs	Vasodilators
Cytotoxic drugs	Etretinate it is teratogenic
Digitalis	Tranquilizers
Dilantin	Drugs of Parkinson's disease
Finasteride it is teratogenic	Acitretin it is teratogenic

- Have you ever had epilepsy?
- Have you ever had a coma or stroke?
- Have you ever had problems with your heart or lungs?
- Have you ever had kidney or blood problems?
- Have you ever had cancer?
- Have you ever had Crohn's disease?
- Have you suffered from bleeding gums?
- Have you suffered from vertigo?
- Have you suffered from mental illness?
- Have you suffered from tuberculosis?
- Have you any reason to believe that you may be infected: By HIV and/or venereal disease: Yes? No?

History of drugs administration of the donor (Table 3.1)

Are you taking or have you taken any of these in the past 72 h? If positive, deferral period for 1 month.

Antibiotics	Steroids	Aspirin	Vaccination	Growth hormone

Aspirin: inhibit platelets

No Deferral
- Immunization with recombinant vaccine
- Primary vaccination against before exposure to disease:
- Diphtheria
- Anthrax
- Cholera
- Hepatitis A
- Influenza
- Injectable polio vaccine
- Lyme disease vaccine

Table 3.2 Showing physical examination report of the donor

Name of the donor				Sex/age	
Weight	BP	Pulse	Temperature	Hemoglobin	ABO/Rh group

Signature of resident doctor	Signature of blood donor
Name of resident doctor	Name of blood donor
Mobile number of the donor	Mobile number of the doctor
Date & time of examination	Date & time of preperation of report

Is there any history of surgery or blood transfusion in the past 6 months?

Major operation	Minor operation	Blood transfusion

For Women Donors:
Are you pregnant?

Do you have a child, <1 year old? Yes/No

Have you ever been pregnant, miscarried, or had an abortion? (For female plasma and platelet donors) Yes/No

Are you rape victims? Deferral

Breastfeeding: Defer till baby is on breastfeeding.

Would you like to be informed about any abnormal test result at the address furnished by you? Yes/No

Lifestyle Questionnaires
The following questions are lifestyle-related questions:

In the past 6 months, have you had a tattoo?

In the past 6 months, have you had skin or ear piercing?

In the past 6 months, have you had acupuncture?

In the past 6 months, have you had electrolysis?

In the past 6 months, have you had an injury from a needle or come in contact with someone else's blood?

In the past 12 months, have you taken illegal steroids with a needle?

In the past 12 months, have you had or been treated for syphilis or gonorrhea?

In the past 12 months, have you been in jail or prison?

In the past 12 months, have you used cocaine?

In the past 12 months, have you had sex with a sex trade worker or anyone else who has taken money or drugs for sex?

In the past 12 months, have you had sex with anyone who has ever taken illegal drugs with a needle?

In the past 12 months, have you had sex with a man who, in the past 12 months, had sex with another man? (Female)

In the past 2 months, have you had sex with another man? (Male)

In the past 12 months, have you had sex with anyone who has HIV/AIDS or has tested positive for HIV/AIDS virus?

At any time since 1977, have you taken money or drugs for sex?

Have you ever taken illegal drugs with a needle even one time?

Have you used intranasal cocaine?

Have you, in your past or present job, taken care of or handled monkeys or their body fluids?

Have you read and understood all the information presented and answered all the questions truthfully? As any incorrect statement or concealment may affect your health or may harm the recipient? Yes? No?

After the donor questionnaires is complete and the donor is found to be suitable candidate for blood collection, perform the physical examination of the donor (Table 3.2).

3.5 Consent Letter from the Donor

I have today read and understand the information provided to me by information booklet for donors. I have been given the opportunity to ask questions, and they have been answered.

To the best of my knowledge, I am not at the risk of infections or transmitting the infections listed the information booklet.

I have understood that blood donation is a totally voluntary act and no inducement or remuneration has been offered. Donation of blood/components is a medical procedure and that by donating voluntarily.

I understand the nature of donation process and the possible risks associated with this procedure. As mentioned in the information booklet.

My blood will be tested for HIV 1 and HIV 2, Hepatitis B antigen, Hepatitis C antigen, Malaria parasite, and VDRL test, in addition to any other screening tests required to ensure blood safety.

I understand that if my donation gives positive result for any of these tests, I will be informed and asked to participate in a post-test discussion.

I agree to blood bank hospital holding information about me, my donation, and my health, to contact my doctor for further information.

I give my blood to blood bank to be used for the benefit of patients. This may be direct transfusion to a patient or for the purpose as explained to me.

I prohibit any information provided by me or about my donation to be disclosed to any individual or government agency without any prior permission.

Signature of the Donor

Date & time

Process of blood donation: Donating blood is a simple, safe, and rewarding experience that usually only takes 10–20 min. In blood donation, a pint of whole blood has been taken, and then the blood is separated into its components: red cells, plasma, and platelets.

It includes a closed collection system with a sterile blood collection bag containing anticoagulant, with an integrally attached tube and needle.

Identify and prepare the donor: Ask the donor to state his full name and label the donor name on blood collection bag, pilot tubes, and donor record register. Ensure the blood collection bag is of the correct type.

Ask donor to lie down on bleeding table and make sure he is relaxed and comfortable.

Find out the bleeding site at the bend of the elbow. Palpate the area, locate a vein of a good size that is visible, straight, and clear. The vein should be visible without applying the tourniquet.

Apply a tourniquet or blood pressure cuff inflated to 40–60 mmHg.

Ask the donor to form a fist so that the veins are more prominent.

Release the tourniquet and disinfect the venipuncture site by using spirit, or 70% isopropyl alcohol, for 30 s. Allow it to dry completely. Do not touch the site after disinfection.

Perform venipuncture with a 16 gauze needle. Anchor the needle and tubing with an adhesive tape. Ask the donor to open and close the first slowly every 10–15 s during collection to have rapid flow of blood from the vein. In thin veins, use 18–20 gauze needles.

Release the tourniquet when the blood flow is established or after 2 min, whichever comes first.

Donor monitoring: Look for pallor, sweating, or complaints of feeling faint that may precede fainting, development of a hematoma at the injection site, and changes in blood flow that may indicate the needle has moved in the vein, and needs to be repositioned.

Mix the collected blood gently with the anticoagulant, either manually or by continuous mechanical mixing, about every 30 s during the donation.

When required, volume of blood has been collected (300–400 mL), which together with 80 mL of ACD solution gives about 400–500 mL or one unit of blood, clamp the tubing, release the tourniquet and object from the fist of hand. It will take approximately 10 min for the collection of blood.

When the required amount of blood is collected, before the needle has been removed from the vein, and trapped blood is drained into the pilot tubes or vials (with or without anticoagulant) delivering 2–4 mL each in tubes. To facilitate the process, clamp the bleeding tube and remove the other end of the bleeding set from the bottle and hold it at a higher level than the pilot tube. Then release the forceps and collect the blood trapped in the bleeding tube into the pilot tube. Draw the needle from the blood bag and put 5–10 mL of sample into the pilot tube or vial.

Now remove the needle from the vein. This procedure can be followed only when the amount of blood held in the clamped blood collecting set is sufficient for both pilot tubes for laboratory testing.

Alternatively when the required amount of blood is collected, before the needle has been removed from the vein, draw the needle from the blood bag set and put 5–10 mL of samples into the pilot tubes or vials.

Now label pilot tube or vials with the same number as that on the main blood bags and label them.

After withdrawal of needle place an alcohol swab over the puncture site. Ask the donor to press the arm held straight up in an extended position. This position gives better pressure and occlusion of the vein than by holding the cotton swab in the flexed elbow. In case if bleeding or bruising appears under the skin, apply a cold pack periodically to the bruised area during the first 24 h, then warm, moist heat intermittently.

Now promptly remove the airway needle from the blood collecting set, and replace the cap after applying a 70% alcohol swab on the open area.

Finally, tally the numbers on the blood bag with donor slip, record book, and the ones on the pilot tubes.

3.5.1 Blood Volume Monitoring

The most efficient way of measuring the blood volume in plastic bags is by weight. The mean weight of 1 mL of blood is 1.06 g, and therefore, for example, a unit containing 400 mL of blood should weigh 400 × 1.06 g plus the weight of the pack(s) and the anticoagulant.

Label the unit of blood as per international regulations as follows (Table 3.3):

Donor care after blood donation: Ask the donor to remain in the chair and relax for 10–12 min

Inspect the venipuncture site; if it is not bleeding, apply a bandage to the site; if it is bleeding, apply further pressure.

Ask the donor to sit up slowly and ask how he is feeling.

Table 3.3 Showing blood group bottle label

Type of blood group	Color of label
O	Blue
A	Yellow
B	Pink
AB	White

Before the donor leaves the donation room, ensure that the person can stand up without dizziness and without drop in blood pressure and strong enough to leave.

Offer the donor hot tea or coffee and some biscuits.

Donor should be given a card with post-donation advice. It is important to keep this card for reference purposes.

Store the blood unit at 2–4 °C. If the blood is collected outside of the laboratory, use ice packs and send the blood promptly to the blood bank.

Enjoy the feeling of accomplishment knowing you are helping to save lives of someone you love.

Take a selfie with blood bank staff or simply share your good deed with friends. It may inspire them to become future blood donors.

Post-donation Instructions

Provide telephone number of doctor if the need arises.

Take liquid diet more than usual in the next 4 h.

Do not smoke for 48 h.

Do not drink alcohol for next 3 days.

Do not take alcoholic drinks for the next 48 h.

After the donor is sent home, monitoring by family member can be done with instructions to promptly seek medical attention from the same hospital where the blood was donated or from the nearest competent donor should donor condition change.

Double red cell donation: Allows donating twice the amount of red blood cells than normally would during a whole blood donation (Table 3.4).

Donor reaction, adverse effect, and its management: Although the blood donation is usually safe and uncomplicated, occasionally donor may experience adverse reactions during or after blood donation; but they are usually harmless.

Table 3.4 Showing blood collection record sheet

Date	Technician job				
Bottle number	Donor name	ABO group	Rh group	Date of collection	Expiry date
1960		O	+ve		
1961		B	+ve		
1962		A	−ve		
1963		O	+ve		
1964		AB	+ve		

Remove or deflate tourniquet and withdraw the needle and discontinue blood collection.

Syncope fainting or vasovagal reaction: Major manifestation is slow heart rate below 60/min as opposed to hypovolemic shock in which heart rate is more than 100 beats/min.

Causes: pain at the site of needle insertion

Management

Elevate the legs: (Trendelenburg position) by placing pillows under the feet, legs, or thigh so that the legs are above head. It will increase blood flow to brain.

Loosen tight clothings.

Ensure adequate airway.

Administer inhalation of aromatic spirit of ammonia.

Apply cold compresses to donor's head.

Check the BP, pulse, and respiratory rate until donor recover.

Aromatic spirit of ammonia: (commercial name aromatic ammonia spirit by Humco.) It contains active compound ammonium carbonate in conjunction with lavender oil or eucalyptus oil.

The inhalant should be held about four inches away from the nostrils and the vapor slowly inhaled until the patient awakens.

Keep aromatic ammonia spirit away from the eyes and skin.

Tetany cause and management: apprehension caused by sight of blood and may cause hyperventilation. Anxiety and deep breathing may cause the excited donor to loose excess of carbon dioxide, which may result in tetany, characterized by muscular spasms due to hyperventilation. The donor is asked to breath into a paper bag which gives prompt relief. Do not give oxygen.

Management of Nausea and Vomiting:

Make the donor comfortable.

Ask the donor to breath slowly and deeply.

Turn the donor's head to one side to avoid aspiration of vomitus, if donor vomits, provide suitable receptacle and towel to clean.

Hematoma:

Deflate the blood pressure cuff. Ask the donor to open the fist and withdraw the needle.

Place sterile gauze over the hematoma and apply digital pressure for few minutes.

Raise the arm and apply cold compression at the venipuncture site for 5 min.

Do not use aspirin to control pain as it may cause further bleeding from the puncture site.

Convulsions and its management: true convulsions are rare, in case if they occur: Prevent the donor from injuring himself by placing tongue blade between the teeth and tongue, ensure adequate airway.

Allergic reaction: with adhesive tape or antiseptic solution used for sterilization of venipuncture site. Rx antiallergic drugs

Identification of Collected Blood:

It is done by (1) blood collection record book, (2) label on blood collection bottle, (3) pilot tube.

3.5.2 Blood Safety Begins with a Healthy Donor

Blood bags: Blood bags first invented by Dr Carl Waldemar Walter, a surgeon in Harvard medical school. Walter has been called "a pioneer in the transfusion and storage of blood bank." He is also credited with founding one of the world first blood banks.

Whole blood is collected currently in containers manufactured from polyolefin or polyvinyl chloride (PVC) that is thinner or plasticized with different compounds such as Triethylhexyl trimellitate and butyryl trihexyl citrate. These bags provide nearly twice the oxygen permeability of first-generation Diethylhexyl phthalate plasticized PVC containers and also maintain pH more than 6 for better platelet survival and function.

Box 3.2: Showing Types of Blood Bags

Single blood bag
Double blood bag
Triple blood bag
Quadruple blood bag
Cord blood collection bag
Blood transferor bags
Top and bottom bags with leukocyte filters

Blood bags are designed for the collection, processing, and storage of whole blood and blood components. They help in providing aseptic conditions for the separation of blood components. It acts as a closed system reducing the chances of contamination.

Quality of blood bags: Blood bags are made up of high molecular weight PVC to ensure better tensile strength and weld strength. Validated sterilization process is monitored by automatically with data logger which confirms the product sterility. Triple filtration of anticoagulant is done and is filled in the bags.

Safety features of blood bags: Needle injury protector provides shielding of needle on withdrawal from vein.

Predonation bags (PDB): It is a constant feature in all blood bags. It diverts 10–30 mL of initial blood, and it reduces the risk of bacterial sepsis (Box 3.2).

Single blood bag: It is used for 250–450 mL of whole blood collection. It contains CPDA 1 solution

Double blood bag: It is also used for the whole blood collection and separation of plasma and red cells

Triple blood bag with SAGM: It is used for whole blood collection and separation of blood components—red cells, plasma, and platelets. The primary bag contains CPD, and one satellite bag contains SAGM.

Quadruple blood bag: It comes with SAGM for whole blood collection and separation for three different blood components (red cells, plasma, and platelets) through the buffy coat method. It is valid for 5 days of platelet storage.

Cord blood collection bag: It has a collection capacity of 200 mL of blood with 22 mL of CPD solution in the collection bag + 8 mL in the rinsing pouch. It is suitable for caesarean section deliveries.

Blood transfer bags: For use with blood bag for transfer or pooling of blood or blood components. They are available in 150 mL, 300 mL, 400 mL, 600 mL, 150 mL, and 50 mL capacity for pediatric use.

Top and bottom bags with leukocyte filters: Top and bottom penta blood bags with leukocyte filter used for whole blood collection and separation of three different blood components (leukocyte depleted red cells, plasma, and platelets). The primary bag contains CPD solution, and one satellite bag is attached to a leukocyte filter which comes with SAGM solution for red cell preservation. Platelets are prepared from buffy coat method.

Precautions to be taken: hermetic sealing of the blood bag tubing should be done to ensure sterility of the collected blood. Blood bags and sample tubes should be correctly labeled. Manufacturing date and expiry date of the blood bags should be carefully noted. Any blood bag that has leaked should be disposed of immediately.

Do not write donor name on blood bags or samples (Table 3.5).

Autologous blood bags: They are available from single to quadruple bag systems from 250 mL to 450 mL capacity with lure connection and leukocyte filter. The bags integrated flap label for patient identification and other details.

3.5.2.1 Red Cell Anticoagulant and Preservative Used in Blood Bags

Citrate: Calcium is the chelating agent. It prevents coagulation by interfering with calcium-dependent steps in the coagulation cascade.

Dextrose: The dextrose provide nutrient for red cells and support the generation of ATP by glycolysis thus enhancing red cells viability and extending shelf life.

Acid–citrate–dextrose: It contains citric acid, sodium citrate, and dextrose. It has a shelf

Table 3.5 Showing types of blood bags with volume

Type	Volume	Anticoagulant
Single volume	250 mL	35 mL CPDA 1
	350 mL	49 mL CPDA1
	450 mL	63 mL CPDA 1
Double blood bag for plasma + red cells	350 mL	49 mL CPDA1
	450 mL	63 mL CPDA 1
Triple blood bag for plasma, red cells, and platelets	350 mL	49 mL CPDA1+ 80 mL SAGM
	450 mL	63 mL CPDA1+ 63 mL CPD+ 100 mL SAGM
Quadruples bag plasma + red cells + platelets + cryoPPT	350 mL	49 mLCPD+ 80 mL SAGM+ 63 mL CPDA1
	450 mL	63 mL CPD+ 100 mL SAGM
Triple bags for plasma + red cells + Buffy coat	350 mL	49 mL CPD+ 80 mL SAGM
	450 mL	63 mL CPD+ 100 mL AS1
Quadruple red cells + plasma + platelets + buffy coat	450 mL	63 mL CPD+ 100 mL SAGM

life of 21 days. It is now no longer use for red cells preservation, as other solutions are available with extended shelf life of red cells. Its acid pH does not help in maintaining 2,3-DPG levels. It is used in apheresis procedure.

3.5.3 Citrate-Phosphate-Dextrose

Alkaline pH helps in maintaining 2,3-DPG level.

Shelf life of red cells is extended to 28 days.

CPD is now most commonly used.

3.5.4 Citrate-Phosphate-Dextrose-Adenine-1 (CPDA-1)

Citrate phosphate dextrose adenine solution was developed in 1968 and shown to permit whole blood storage for 5 weeks. The citrate prevents coagulation by binding or chelating to calcium; phosphate acts as a buffer and, hence, maintains the pH of the blood. Dextrose serves as substrate for the blood cells, while adenine maintains high ATP level in the RBC. Most blood collection bags (adult) contain 63 mL CPDA anticoagulant which is sufficient to ant coagulate and ensure the viability of blood cells in 450 mL ± 10% blood for up to 28–35 days when the blood is stored at 2–8 °C.

Addition of adenine is associated with improved synthesis of ATP, allowing longer shelf life of 35 days.

3.5.5 Other Solutions

Adsol (AS-1)

Nutricel (AS-3)

Optiso (AS-5)

Rejuvenile solution contains
Pyruvate
Inosine
Glucose
Phosphate with or without adenine

3.5.6 Saline-Adenine-Glucose-Mannitol (SAGM)

After taking blood donation in CPD and separating red cells from plasma and platelets, SAGM is added to the packed red cells. The resulting red cells have flow characteristics equivalent to plasma-reduced blood and a storage life of 35–42 days.

Other advantage is by removing maximum amount of plasma from blood for the manufacture of factor VIII and albumin.

SAGM additive solution provides optimum red cell viability.

Sodium chloride provides isotonicity.

Adenine maintains ATP for red cell viability.

Glucose supports red cell metabolism (nutrition).

Mannitol helps reduce red cell lysis.

TOTM (trioctyl trimellitate) plasticized platelet transfer bag with sufficient gas permeability is suitable for extended storage of viable platelets for approximately 5 days at 25 °C.

Table 3.6 Showing anticoagulant used in blood bags

Anticoagulant type	Shelf life
ACD (acidified citrate–dextrose) whole blood	21 days
CPD (citrate–phosphate–dextrose)whole blood	28 days
Citrate–phosphate–dextrose–adenine (CPDA)whole blood	35 days
Saline–adenine–glucose–mannitol (SAGM) whole blood	42 days
Packed red cells	42 days

Anticoagulant citrate–phosphate–dextrose (CPD) solution with an integral container of additive solution (AS-1) and an integral Leukoflex MTL1-WB Leukocyte Reduction Filter for Whole Blood (Table 3.6).

Further Reading

A Code of Ethics for Blood Donation and Transfusion. Amsterdam: International Society of Blood Transfusion; 2006. Archived from http://www.isbt-web.org/fileadmin/user_upload/ISBT_Code_of_Ethics/Code_of_ethics_new_logo_-_feb_2011.pdf

Aide-mémoire. Blood safety. Geneva: World Health Organization; 2002. Archived from http://www.who.int/bloodsafety/publications/who_bct_02_03/en/index.html

Becker CD, Stichtenoth DO, Wichmann MG, Schaefer C, Szinicz L. Blood donors on medication–an approach to minimize drug burden for recipients of blood products and to limit deferral of donors. Transfusion Med Hemother. 2009;36(2):107–13.

Blood Donation: What to Expect. Mayo Clinic. Archived from the original on December. 2008;4. Archived from https://www.mayoclinic.org/tests-procedures/blood-donation/about/pac-20385144

Blood Donor Information Leaflet. Irish Blood Transfusion Service. Archived from the original on November 19, 2007. Archived from https://www.scotblood.co.uk/giving-blood/publications/giving-blood-donor-information-leaflet/

Blood Products Advisory Committee, 12 December 2003. Archived from the original on November 8, 2008. Archived from https://www.fda.gov/advisory-committees/blood-vaccines-and-other-biologics/blood-products-advisory-committee

Brecher ME. AABB technical manual. 15th ed. Bethesda: American Association of Blood Banks; 2005. p. 665–7.

Brooks JP. The rights of blood recipients should supersede any asserted rights of blood donors. Vox sanguinis. 2004;87(4):280–6.

Donating—Frequently Asked Questions. Blood Bank of Alaska. Archived from the original on June 6, 2008. Archived from https://www.bloodbankofalaska.org/wp-content/uploads/2020/05/Convalescent-Plasma-FAQs.pdf

FDA Regulations on Donor Deferral. US Food and Drug Administration. Archived from the original on May 14, 2008. Archived from https://www.accessdata.fda.gov/scripts/cdrh/cfdocs/cfcfr/CFRSearch.cfm?fr=610.41

Franklin IM. Is there a right to donate blood? Patient rights; donor responsibilities. Transfusion Med. 2007;17(3):161–8.

Guidelines for the Blood Transfusion Services in the United Kingdom: donor selection guidelines. 7th ed. London: UK Blood Transfusion & Tissue Transplantation Services; 2005. Archived from http://www.transfusionguidelines.org.uk & http://www.transfusionguidelines.org.uk/index.aspx?Publication=WB

Guidelines for UK Blood Services. UK Blood and Tissue Services. Archived from the original on May 15, 2008. Archived from https://www.nc3rs.org.uk/results-search/all/Guidelines%20for%20UK%20Blood%20Services

Norda A, Behr-Gross M, Heiden E. Risk behaviours having an impact on blood donor management: P-025. Vox Sanguinis. 2011;101:91–2.

Permanent Exclusion Criteria/Dyskwalifikacjastała (in Polish). RCKiK Warszawa. Archived from the original on August 30, 2009. Retrieved 2010-03-03.

Reiss RF. Blood donor well-being: a primary responsibility of blood collection agencies. Ann Clin Lab Sci. 2011;41(1):3–7.

Stichtenoth DO, Deicher HR, Frölich JC. Blood donors on medication. Eur J Clin Pharmacol. 2001;57(6–7):433–40.

World Health Organization. Safe blood and blood products: trainer's guide: World Health Organization; 2002.

World Health Organization. Blood donor selection: guidelines on assessing donor suitability for blood donation: World Health Organization; 2012.

World Health Organization. Blood donor counselling. Implementation Guidelines; 2014.

4 Storage of Blood

Transportation of blood after collection falls into three different categories; they are:

- Transportation of donated blood from field, blood camps, and other collection site to processing center or blood bank.
- From the hospital blood bank to a different facility (to another blood bank, clinic or hospital).
- From the blood bank to hospital wards or operating theater.

Transportation of blood from the field (short- or long-distance travel) is done by transport container. The aim of a transport container is to provide a secure controlled temperature environment for blood and components in transit from one location to another.

The temperature of whole blood and red cell components must be kept at +2 to +10 °C during transport, and the specially designed blood transport boxes should be used.

Why store blood at 2–6 °C?

If blood is not stored between +2 and +6 °C, its oxygen-carrying ability is greatly reduced.

Another important reason for storing blood between +2 and +6 °C is to keep the blood unit free from the growth of any bacterial contamination. If blood is stored above +6 °C, the chances of contamination with bacteria increase.

Hold-over time: Defined as the length of time that the temperature remains within the acceptable range when there is a loss of power.

The blood cold chain from collection to transfusion: Donated whole blood or plasma can be stored in the transport box at +20 to +24 °C for 6 hour only.

Table 4.1 Storage and transport conditions for whole blood and red cells

Condition	Temperature (°C)	Storage time
Transport of pre-processed blood	+20 to +24	<5 hours
Storage of pre-processed or processed blood	+2 to +6	<35 days
Transport of processed blood	+2 to +10	<24 hours

4.1 Essential Features of a Whole Blood and Component Transport Container

Transport container is made up of an insulated box that, when sealed, provides a space that is isolated from the external (ambient) environment. The inside temperature of the box is controlled by efficient insulation, and it prevents from changing as a result of ambient temperature. In spite of the good insulation, isolation from external temperature is never absolute, and

P. S. Ajmani, *Immunohematology and Blood banking*, https://doi.org/10.1007/978-981-15-8435-0_4

gradually, over time, the temperature within the container will equilibrate to the external temperature. Placing frozen coolant inside the container extends the time taken for this process, as it absorbs heat already in the container, or that from the environment that is able to penetrate the insulation. The internal environment of the container attempts to cool to the melting point of the frozen coolant placed in it, to reduce the temperature of freshly donated blood from body temperature (+37 °C) to +22 ± 2 °C within 4 hour of collection. After this initial cooling, requiring considerable heat to be transferred to the coolant pack, the container is expected to maintain the temperature within that range for up to 24 h. To achieve this purpose, the warm blood is placed directly onto frozen coolant plates or individually against frozen coolant bricks.

The use of insulated blood transportation boxes on motorcycles (provided they are securely installed) may be shown to be acceptable in terms of maintaining acceptable transit temperatures.

Reusable containers are usually made of formed plastic or fiberglass filled with high-density polyurethane foam. They are easy to clean (no ridges) and store (optimum width, length, and height for stacking). The container should be robust and able to withstand repeated handling during transportation. The container should have a unique ID number, preferably eye readable and bar-coded, which can be recorded for tracking purposes. Transport containers used for this purpose should not hold more than 10–15 units of whole blood. Keeping the quantity low ensures that loaded containers are of manageable weight for blood collection personnel to handle. Variable quantities of blood components will require the use of different size insulated containers and varying quantities of coolant. It is advisable to use a "space filler" such as shredded paper in a plastic bag, sponge sheets, or bubble plastic to fill air space if the container is not full. This will prevent product movement during transit and will also result in improved temperature maintenance. The insulated boxes need to be made of lightweight but durable material to facilitate movement, to minimize transport costs, and to guard against damage in transit.

4.1.1 Characteristics of Coolant Packs Used in Transportation of Blood

The coolant packs used should have a melting point of approximately 0 to +2 °C. They must be frozen in a freezer set between −10 and −20 °C immediately prior to use. Care should be taken to ensure that these coolant packs are not too cold; ideally they should be frozen solid but close to melting point at time of use. To prevent accidental freezing of red cells, especially those located near the outer plastic of the blood bags, an appropriate insulating material such as foam sheeting or corrugated plastic must be placed between the coolant packs and the blood bags.

4.1.2 Temperature Control by Ice Packs

The melting point of frozen water is 0 °C. At this temperature, ice stops getting warmer and begins to melt, losing its rigid shape and transforming into water (known as phase change). The energy (heat) used to transform a certain mass of frozen ice into a liquid, without changing its temperature, is called the latent heat of melting. Water requires a lot of heat energy (latent heat) when changing from solid phase (ice) to liquid phase (water) and will absorb as much heat energy in converting from a solid to a liquid, as it will take to warm the resulting water to about +80 °C.

Containers and coolant packs used for this purpose are required to maintain the temperature of previously stored (cooled) blood between +1 and +10 °C during transportation. Provision for safe transportation of a minimum of one red cell concentrate (or one whole blood) and a maximum of approximately 40 red cell concentrates (or 20 whole blood) per container should be made when designing a system.

Following the collection of blood, it should be kept at a temperature of 2–8 °C. Care should be taken so as not to allow the red cells to freeze, as this will cause lysis. A temperature of 4 ± 2 °C is considered to be ideal, but this is difficult to maintain during transportation. To maintain the desired temperature, place the blood bag in wet ice in a waterproof container (plastic bag) placed in sturdy, well-insulated cardboard or Styrofoam plastic containers (polystyrene). If melting ice is used to achieve an appropriate storage temperature, it should not come into direct contact with the components. Dead air space in packaging containers should be minimized.

The cooling material ice should be placed above the container with blood. This is done in order to take advantage of the downward movement of cool air. Considering the hot weather of India and other developing countries, during hot trips it is advisable to keep the ice and the blood bag in direct contact with each other. In a very hot weather, the ice may be placed both above and below the blood bag. Any air space or layer of cardboard between ice and blood bag may act as internal insulator, preventing the ice from adequately protecting the blood from high atmospheric temperature.

Wet ice only 0 °C fresh (crushed ice that is not frozen solid or cubed ice with a glistening or melting surface) is commonly used for short-distance travel, but cubed ice is considered to be better option than chipped ice for long-distance travel shipments because it melts slowly. The volume of ice and blood should be equal in long-distance shipments. Do not use dry ice for the shipment of blood; it may cause skin burns. Use dry ice for only frozen blood products.

With proper insulation blood container cases containing blood being kept in the cold room when not in use, it will give a satisfactory "hold-over" temperature below 10 °C for 12 hour and possibly over 24 hour depending on the ambient temperature. After the blood has arrived at the blood bank laboratory, it is safer to check the temperature by keeping the thermometer between the blood bag and plastic bag. If the temperature of blood bag is above 10 °C, it should not be stored, but may be released for immediate use. Always discard hemolyzed blood. Good organization and team work is necessary for reducing mishandling of donor blood.

The problem of blood transportation is not only a matter of concern between the blood collection point and the blood bank but also within the hospital. There is a time gap between the issue of the blood or its components and giving of transfusion to the patient. During this period, the blood is most often kept at room temperature which varies widely, during different seasons.

4.2 Visual Inspection of the Collected Blood

Before placing the unit in the refrigerator, it should be inspected for:

- Integrity of the pack by checking for leaks at the ports and seams.
- Any evidence of hemolysis at the interface between plasma and red cells.
- Any evidence of discoloration of the red cells.
- Presence of small and large clots in the red cells.

If there is any evidence of the above, the unit should not be used and discarded.

Hospital ward refrigerator: In case the transfusion cannot be commenced within 20 min, the blood may be stored in an approved and monitored blood storage refrigerator in the hospital ward until required for transfusion.

Transit condition within the hospital must be controlled and properly monitored by the blood bank.

The unused blood should be returned within 30 min, because the blood stored at 2–6 °C warms up to 10 °C or above within 30 min at room temperature. In hot weather, the time between the issue of blood and return of the unused blood should be further reduced.

4.3 Documentation Along with the Transport Container

All transport containers should be appropriately labeled and should be secure and protect components and samples from damage during transit.

Documentation should accompany components in transit to permit their identification.

Donations from which it is intended to prepare platelets should be transported in conditions that ensure the surface temperature of the blood packs does not drop below 20 °C.

The following steps have to be carried out while receiving the blood from a distant site blood collection camp or similar collection center.

Compare the time the blood was received in the blood bank with the time of the first donation at the clinic. The time interval should not exceed 8 hour if the blood is to be used to make labile components such as fresh frozen plasma.

Check the actual blood packs received against the donor clinic records, i.e., the donor clinic register and the donor enrolment forms received.

Check that the donation number on the sample attached to the unit matches that of the blood pack. Check the temperature of the blood packs on receipt.

Any signs suggesting leak in the pack, air in the pack, or that it has already been opened should be discarded.

In the case of frozen plasma, see for the cracks in the plasma packs and any evidence of the plasma thawing.

Platelet swirling phenomenon, due to the light-scattering effect of normal platelets in movement, can be used as a quality control procedure, or as a routine check before issue.

The following guidelines should be used for non-transfusion of blood units:

- All blood units which have tested positive for infectious agents.
- Unsuitable products, such as under- and over-weight blood packs or those where the temperature range has not been maintained.
- Blood units whose shelf life has been expired.
- Blood returned unused but unsuitable for reissue.
- Blood packs in which leaks have been detected. There should be a mechanism in place for reporting.

4.4 Transport of Blood Components from One Station to Another

It can be done easily to transfer components like red cells, FFP, and platelets, provided that the transport has been validated for use.

The following information should be provided by the supplying hospital:

- Guarantee that the units have been appropriately stored prior to dispatch.
- The time the transport box is validated for—by component.
- The time of dispatch from the sending hospital.

Concern about blood product's temperature begins when they are dispatched from the blood bank to different wards within the hospital and placed out of refrigerator in ambient temperature for an undetermined length of time.

Blood components should be transported under conditions which are as close as possible to their specific storage requirements to the hospital, provided each component type ensuring core temperature is maintained, specifically for the number of components to be transferred and the time taken to transfer.

It should be noted that, occasionally, red cell components are issued before they have been cooled to their storage temperature (4 ± 2 °C). In such circumstances, it may be neither possible nor necessary to maintain the transport temperature within the range 2–10 °C, and local judgment should be exercised.

A copy of the signed and annotated dispatch note (either paper or an electronic equivalent acceptable to the quality director) should be returned to the blood supplier blood bank.

It is strongly recommended all records pertaining to donor and donation identity be entered and maintained in an electronic format which can be accessed readily by approved and qualified

Table 4.2 Showing blood disposal log

Reason for disposal					
Date	Blood bag ID	Temp	Time (30 min rule)	Expiry date	Comments

personnel and in a manner which preserves donor confidentiality in accordance with legal requirements. Machine-readable systems for identifying donors and donation derivatives are also recommended. Initial documentation—for example, on session records—may be taken manually and archived for the required period in law, with relevant portions transcribed electronically whenever convenient operationally (Table 4.2).

Storage of blood: for storage of whole blood and its different components, the following equipment are required:

- **Blood bank refrigerator(s)**: to hold blood undergoing processing before it is released for use.
- **Blood plasma freezer(s)**: for storing prepared plasma components, like FFP and cryoprecipitate.
- **Platelet agitator(s) with built-in incubators**: for storing platelet concentrates (+20 to +24 °C).

4.5 Temperature Recording Devices and Alarms

Blood collected from the donor should be stored at a temperature between 2 and 4 °C in blood bank refrigerators. After collection from donor, blood should be processed for component separation within 6 h.

Blood can be stored in walk-in cold rooms; in freestanding, reach-in refrigerated cabinets; or in refrigerators on vehicle. The installation requirements of walk-in cold rooms and reach-in refrigerators are identical. The refrigerator should maintain a temperature between 2 and 4 °C. A blower circulates the air, so that the same temperature is maintained through the refrigerated space. A dial-type thermometer indicating the air temperature with −20 to 20 °C in the refrigerator should be placed in a prominent position. There should be an audible and visible alarm system that will give the earliest possible indication of any undesirable change in the air temperature above 4 °C, whether this is due to electrical or mechanical failure, or a careless act of keeping the refrigerator door open. The air temperature fluctuates more rapidly than fluid (blood) stored in containers. Hence the alarm gives sufficient time to protect the blood.

The alarm should not be connected to electrical system. A battery-operated alarm system is recommended.

A permanent record of the actual storage temperature of the blood is of paramount importance. This is done by placing a standard bottle with 500 mL of water within the refrigerator and by immersing a sensor (thermocouple or thermometer bulb) in the water. A 7-day circular chart is preferred to a strip chart (daily) so that the variations can be compared, at a glance, over several days. The recorder should have an independent power supply from the refrigerator and should be mounted on adjoining wall not subject to any vibrations.

All the freestanding blood storage refrigerators should be wired back to a fuse box or distribution board in a permanent way and should not be connected with a switched outlet. This precaution is taken in order to avoid accidental switching off the refrigerator's power supply. It is important to check alarm system periodically; one way to check it is to warm up the sensing device with warm water. The alarm should function when the temperature reaches 4 °C. Similarly, cool the sensing device by dipping in chipped ice, and the alarm should sound when the temperature goes below 1 °C.

4.6 Receipt and Handling of Incoming, Unprocessed Blood and Plasma Derivative

Blood collected from donors, visiting the blood bank clinic, is generally kept at temperature of 22–24 °C until there is enough quantity to process, which largely depends on the blood storage cabinets and centrifuge space.

Blood bank refrigerator is an essential piece of equipment in the immunohematology department and provides safe and convenient storage of whole blood, blood components (pRBCs, and fresh frozen plasma), blood bank reagents, and testing kits. Blood bank refrigerator (BBR) or blood storage refrigerator is a designated temperature-controlled refrigeration equipment specifically designed to store blood bags.

In PHCbi-designed technology, a special compressor is used to provide rapid cooling of 4 °C, having quiet performance with flexible storage capacity and uniformity with microprocessor control. The blood bank refrigerators are available with capacity to store 32, 120, 360, and 720 bags. Blood storage cabinets come in different designs including chest, benchtop, and floor-standing.

The basic model of blood refrigerator is having capacity to store from 40 to 150 bags or more, depending upon quantity and size of blood bags.

Upright refrigerator: Blood bank refrigerators are usually of the "upright type" with glass doors. This is because they are frequently opened to place or retrieve blood packs.

Chest refrigerators: Ice-lined and solar-powered refrigerators are of the chest type and have a cooling fan to ensure air circulation within the cabinet. Ice-lined refrigerators are designed to achieve a relatively longer hold-over temperature because they are used in locations that experience frequent and lengthy power cuts.

4.6.1 Capacity of Refrigerators

The internal capacity of a blood bank refrigerator is measured by number of blood bags stored inside the chamber. Standard models are available in 24, 50, 100, 200, and 300 blood bag capacities. Furthermore, these can be designed in benchtop and floor-standing models.

4.6.2 Temperature Monitoring

In order to monitor accurate temperature of blood refrigerator, digital sensor (PT-100) is dipped in liquid medium. This temperature monitoring system is used to read accurate temperature of blood bags and avoid temperature deviation due to frequent opening and closing of door. Blood bank refrigerator should be provided with a temperature recorder (weekly chart recorder) or programmable logic controller (PLC) memory storage.

4.6.3 Air Circulation and Refrigeration

Blood refrigerator system should have a positive forced air circulation to maintain temperature uniformity at all shelf levels with ±1 °C.

4.6.4 Temperature Controller

Blood storage refrigerator is equipped with three types of digital temperature controller, i.e., PID temp controller, PLC (programmable logic controller)-based temp controllers, and microprocessor-based temp controller in order to maintain preferable temperature accuracy and uniformity. This controller shows both SV (set value) and PV (present value) on the LED screen. Digital temperature (LED) display with 0.1 °C graduation temperature recording device.

Audiovisual Alarms: Blood refrigerator should have audiovisual temperature alarm that is provided in the unit for protection during temperature fluctuations. It should have safety system to ensure secure locking of the door. In addition, battery backup for alarm and temperature recording device with minimum 4 hour battery backup. SMS alerts are sent to user-defined recipients in case of any deviation in temperature breakdown and power failure with provision to connect with central (temperature) monitoring system.

Safe-T-Vue® Temperature-Sensitive Indicators: These are nonreversible indicators designed to attach directly to blood bags during refrigeration, transport, and temporary storage. They are available in 6 and 10 °C. The indicator changes color from white to red when the blood (or other temperature-sensitive product) has reached or exceeded 6 °C. It helps in making decision whether or not blood products, plasma, and RBCs can safely be reissued (Fig. 4.1).

4.6.5 Plasma Storage Freezers

The purpose of a plasma storage freezer is to store plasma for therapeutic use and bulk plasma for transfer to a fractionation facility at temperatures consistently colder than −30 to −40 °C. Freezers require a "defrost cycle" to clear ice from the fan (blower) unit. During the defrost cycle, the temperature in the freezer may rise approximately 5 °C, so in order to maintain a temperature consistently colder than −25 °C, the operating temperature of the freezer should be set at −30 °C or colder. The purpose of a plasma freezer is to provide a maintained freezing temperature of −30 °C or −40 °C for safe storage of fresh frozen plasma, red cells, and cryoprecipitate (Table 4.3).

4.6.5.1 Types of Plasma Storage Freezers

Ultra-low temperature (ULT) freezers: Minus 80 °C lab freezers, also known as ultra-low temperature (ULT) freezers, are designed first and foremost to protect blood products like FFP, cryoprecipitate, and blood samples. They're also designed to maximize storage capacity by offering a range of upright and chest models to accommodate a variety of laboratory footprint requirements. Samples like DNA, RNA, antigens, bacteria, viruses, cell liners, and more are being stored in these freezers. Most ULT freezers operate between −80 and −86 °C.

−40 °C Upright Freezers: Upright free-standing chest-type freezers are commonly used for both small quantity and bulk plasma storage applications. As cold air is heavier than warm, it remains at the bottom of a chest freezer when the top-opening lid is raised, and it is this feature that makes chest-type freezers most suitable.

−40 °C chest freezers: These standard chest freezers, versatile and reliable sample storage for applications requiring a temperature range from −10 to −40 °C, come in a variety of sizes and offer a full range of racking solutions. Storage

Table 4.3 Showing specification of plasma storage freezers

10 to −40 °C temperature range	PID controller for superior accuracy
Capacity up to 25 cu. ft or more	Auto-defrost
User-friendly design	Doors with lock
Audiovisual alarms	Temperature chart recorder
Password protection	CFC-free refrigerant
Separate inner door to prevent cold loss	Caster wheels for easy mobility

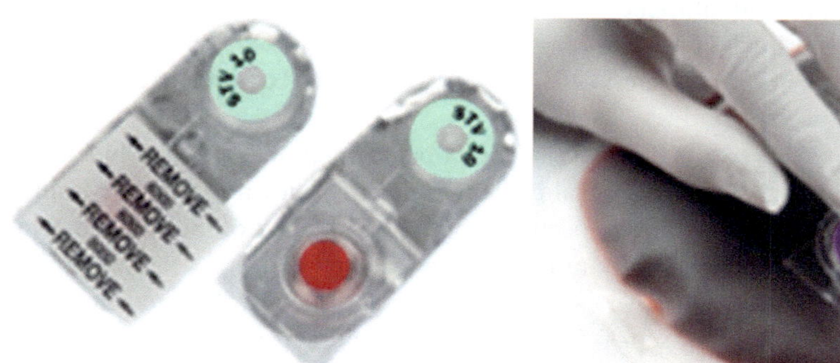

Fig. 4.1 Temperature-sensitive indicators

capacity ranges from 63 to 396 unit boxes to fit blood bank needs.

Blood plasma freezers with −32 and −40 °C are available for plasma storage. The temperature is maintained automatically by an electronic, microprocessor-controlled temperature regulator, even in the event of changing ambient temperatures. Rapid defrosting with thermal and temporal monitoring takes place automatically.

4.6.6 Cold Room for Preservation of Blood

Cold room is providing an area that complies with good laboratory practice (GLP) and a temperature-controlled working environment for good laboratory practice where units of blood are processed or handled in bulk (i.e., sorting of incoming fresh blood, labeling, preparing deliveries, and so on).

Cold rooms or freezer rooms are fixtures built into a blood transfusion center. They vary in size and design and are usually constructed at the same time as the facility is built so that their features may be carefully planned. The purpose of creating a room temperature storage facility is to provide a controlled environment, validated to maintain temperature at +22 ± 2 °C, under all ambient conditions (extreme heat or cold). Freezer rooms are best suited to bulk storage of plasma that is destined for fractionation or large-scale quarantine of plasma in a "donor retest" program or, if properly segregated and labeled, general storage of all these types of plasma.

Such an environment is required **for platelet storage and** storage of crates and trays of fresh blood (less than 24 hour from donation) that are to be processed.

4.6.7 Organization in Storage

Refrigerators in the blood bank must be properly organized. There should be separate areas or separate refrigerators for the following groups:

Unprocessed blood: Blood recently collected from donor and waiting for blood grouping and Rh typing.

Processed blood: This is the group of collected blood whose blood group and type have been determined and available for crossmatching.

Crossmatched blood: This group of blood has been crossmatched with the patient (recipient) for whom the blood was requested. It is now waiting for delivery. Every blood bank must bear the identification of recipient, and the pilot tubes have been separated and stored for future use in case of transfusion reaction.

Crossmatched blood: This is the group of outdated blood, quarantined and waiting for disposal.

The unit must be discarded: should be in continution with if it has been out of the refrigerator for longer than 30 min, if the seal is broken, if there is any sign that the pack has been opened, if there is a sign of hemolysis, and if the temperature is over +10 °C for more than 30 min.

4.7 Disadvantages of Using Blood That Has Not Been Stored Between +2 and +6 °C

Increased risk of disease transmission: Intracellular pathogens (CMV, HTLV) survive in leukocytes present in fresh blood.

Syphilis transmission: *Treponema pallidum* cannot survive >96 hour in stored blood at a temperature of 1–6 °C.

Malaria transmission: Malarial parasite cannot survive >7 hour in stored blood.

4.8 Changes in Stored Blood

It is well documented that certain biochemical changes generally known as **storage lesions** occur during the 35–42 days of blood at temperatures between 1 and 6 °C.

The biochemical structure of the red blood cell (RBC) changes due to anaerobic glycolysis (cellular metabolism), and these changes are relative to the storage period which can affect the efficacy of blood transfusion.

The viability of the red cells decreases up to 25% in 21 days.

Diphosphoglycerate (DPG) level declines, and the free-floating DPG enters into hemoglobin configuration at the oxygen-binding sites, resulting in reduced oxygen-carrying capacity of red cells.

There is increase in potassium level. Normally, potassium is 500 times higher in the cell than in plasma. Lysis of cells releases this cytosolic content into the plasma. There is increased cell lysis that occurs as blood is being stored awaiting transfusion.

There is increase in lactate level and loss of 33% of factor VIII within 48 h.

pH: The decrease in pH during storage of blood is as follows (Table 4.4):

White cells lose their phagocytic property within 4–6 hour of collection and become non-functional after 24 hour of storage.

Few lymphocytes may remain viable even after 3 weeks of storage.

Platelets lose their functional capacity within 24 h.

4.9 Storage of Donor Red Cell Unit Considerations

Addition of AS-1 and AS-3 nutrient increases the storage life of pRBC, or whole blood, up to 42 days.

Posttransfusion recovery pRBCs is 73–83% after storage of 42 days (maximal storage).

High level of ATP is maintained in the stored blood up to the 28th day of storage.

The levels of 2,3-DPG and P50 values may not be fully maintained.

Table 4.4 Showing pH of blood on different days

Day	pH
0 (CPD)	7.40
3 (CPD)	7.20
11 (CPD)	7.0
35 (CPD)	6.84

Decreased recovery and shortened half-life of pRBCS or whole blood may increase transfusion requirements and increase the risk of iron overload.

The current recommended practice is to use red cells stored in additive solutions for <2 weeks old.

Further Reading

AABB. Recovered plasma. Archived from http://www.aabb.org/Search/Pages/results.aspx?k=recovered%20plasma.

Abdel-Wahab OI, Healy B, Dzik WH. Effect of fresh-frozen plasma transfusion on prothrombin time and bleeding in patients with mild coagulation abnormalities. Transfusion. 2006;46(8):1279–85.

Australian Red Cross Blood Service. Giving blood -> What to expect. Archived from the original on 29 Aug 2007. Retrieved 6 Oct 2007.

British Committee for Standards in Haematology, Blood Transfusion Task Force. Guidelines for the use of platelet transfusions. Br J Haematol. 2003;122(1):10.

British Committee for Standards in Haematology, Blood Transfusion Task Force (Duguid J, Chairman), O'Shaughnessy DF, Atterbury C, Bolton Maggs P, Murphy M, Thomas D, Yates S, Williamson LM. Guidelines for the use of fresh-frozen plasma, cryoprecipitate and cryosupernatant. Br J Haematol. 2004a;126(1):11–28.

British Committee for Standards in Haematology, Blood Transfusion Task Force (Duguid J, Chairman), O'Shaughnessy DF, Atterbury C, Bolton Maggs P, Murphy M, Thomas D, Yates S, Williamson LM. Guidelines for the use of fresh-frozen plasma, cryoprecipitate and cryosupernatant. Br J Haematol. 2004b;126(1):11–28.

BS/EN/ISO 3826-3. Plastics collapsible containers for human blood and blood components—Part 3: Blood bag systems with integrated features.

Carino G, Tsapenko A, Sweeney J. Fresh frozen plasma use before line insertion in critically-ill patients with coagulation abnormalities. Crit Care Med. 2009;37(12):A468.

Carson JL, Grossman BJ, Kleinman S, Tinmouth AT, Marques MB, Fung MK, Holcomb JB, Illoh O, Kaplan LJ, Katz LM, Rao SV. Red blood cell transfusion: a clinical practice guideline from the AABB. Ann Intern Med. 2012a;157(1):49–58.

Carson JL, Grossman BJ, Kleinman S, Tinmouth AT, Marques MB, Fung MK, Holcomb JB, Illoh O, Kaplan LJ, Katz LM, Rao SV. Red blood cell transfusion: a clinical practice guideline from the AABB. Ann Intern Med. 2012b;157(1):49–58.

Carson JL, Guyatt G, Heddle NM, Grossman BJ, Cohn CS, Fung MK, Gernsheimer T, Holcomb JB, Kaplan

LJ, Katz LM, Peterson N. Clinical practice guidelines from the AABB: red blood cell transfusion thresholds and storage. JAMA. 2016;316(19):2025–35.

College of American Pathologists. Easy does it—showing caution with RBC transfusions. 2009. Archived from http://www.captodayonline.com/Archives/0409/0409d_easy_does_it.html.

Commission of European Communities. Directive 2002/98/EC of The European Parliament and Council of 27th January 2003 and daughter directives. Setting standards of safety and quality for collecting, processing, testing, storage and distribution of human blood and blood components.

Cooper ES, Bracey AW, Horvath AE, Shanberge JN, Simon TL, Yawn DH. Practice parameter for the use of fresh-frozen plasma, cryoprecipitate, and platelets. JAMA. 1994;271(10):777–81.

Daniels G. Other blood groups. In: Roback JD, Grossman BJ, Harris T, Hillyer CD, editors. Technical manual. 17th ed. Bethesda, MD: AABB; 2011. p. 433.

Dzik WH, Blajchman MA, Fergusson D, Hameed M, Henry B, Kirkpatrick AW, Korogyi T, Logsetty S, Skeate RC, Stanworth S, MacAdams C. Clinical review: Canadian National Advisory Committee on Blood and Blood Products-Massive Transfusion Consensus Conference 2011: report of the panel. Crit Care. 2011;15(6):242.

EN ISO 3826-1. Plastics collapsible containers for human blood and blood components–Part 1: Conventional containers.

EN ISO 3826-2:2008. Plastics collapsible containers for human blood and blood components. Part 2: Graphic symbols for use on labels and instruction leaflets. Archived from https://www.iso.org/standard/45611.html.

EN ISO 980:2008. Graphical symbols for use in the labelling of medical devices. Archived from https://www.iso.org/standard/69081.html.

Estcourt L, Birchall J, Allard S, Bassey SJ, Hersey P, Kerr JP, Mumford AD, Stanworth SJ, Tinegate H. Guidelines for the use of platelet transfusions. Br J Haematol. 2016;176(3):365–94.

European Directorate for the Quality of Medicines. Guide to the preparation, use and quality assurance of blood components.

Goodnough LT, Levy JH, Murphy MF. Concepts of blood transfusion in adults. Lancet. 2013;381(9880):1845–54.

Gottschall J, editor. Blood transfusion therapy: a physician's handbook. Bethesda, MD: AABB; 2005.

Greeno E, McCullough J, Weisdorf D. Platelet utilization and the transfusion trigger: a prospective analysis. Transfusion. 2007;47(2):201–5.

Haas FLJM, van Rhenen DJ, de Vries RRP, Overbeeke MAM, Novotny VMJ, Henny CP. Blood transfusion guideline. Utrecht, Netherlands: Institute for Healthcare Improvement; 2011. Archived from http://www.isbtweb.org/fileadmin/user_upload/blood-transfusion-guideline.pdf.

Hillyer C, Hillyer KL, Strobl F, Jefferies L, Silberstein L, editors. Handbook of transfusion medicine. Cambridge, MA: Academic; 2001.

Holland LL, Brooks JP. Toward rational fresh frozen plasma transfusion: the effect of plasma transfusion on coagulation test results. Am J Clin Pathol. 2006;126(1):133–9.

Klein HG, Anstee DJ. Mollison's blood transfusion in clinical medicine. Hoboken, NJ: Wiley; 2014.

Kumar A, Mhaskar R, Grossman BJ, Kaufman RM, Tobian AA, Kleinman S, Gernsheimer T, Tinmouth AT, Djulbegovic B, AABB Platelet Transfusion Guidelines Panel. Platelet transfusion: a systematic review of the clinical evidence. 2015 Transfusion; 55(5):1116-1127.

National Institutes of Health Consensus Development Conference Statement. Fresh frozen plasma: indications and risks. NIH Consens Statement. 1984;5(5):4. PMid: 6395009. Archived from https://consensus.nih.gov/1984/1984FrozenPlasma045html.htm.

O'Shaughnessy DF, Atterbury C, Bolton Maggs P, Murphy M, Thomas D, Yates S, Williamson LM, British Committee for Standards in Haematology BTTF. Guidelines for the use of fresh-frozen plasma, cryoprecipitate and cryosupernatant. Br J Haematol. 2004;126(1):11–28.

Padhi S, Kemmis-Betty S, Rajesh S, Hill J, Murphy MF. Blood transfusion: summary of NICE guidance. BMJ. 2015;351:h5832.

Retter A, Wyncoll D, Pearse R, Carson D, McKechnie S, Stanworth S, Allard S, Thomas D, Walsh T, British Committee for Standards in Haematology. Guidelines on the management of anaemia and red cell transfusion in adult critically ill patients. Br J Haematol. 2013;160(4):445–64.

Riley W, Smalley B, Pulkrabek S, Clay ME, McCullough J. Using lean techniques to define the platelet (PLT) transfusion process and cost-effectiveness to evaluate PLT dose transfusion strategies. Transfusion. 2012;52(9):1957–67.

Robinson S, Harris A, Atkinson S, Atterbury C, Bolton-Maggs P, Elliott C, Hawkins T, Hazra E, Howell C, New H, Shackleton T. The administration of blood components: a British Society for Haematology Guideline. Transfus Med. 2018;28(1):3–21.

Seifried E, Klueter H, Weidmann C, Staudenmaier T, Schrezenmeier H, Henschler R, Greinacher A, Mueller MM. How much blood is needed? Vox Sang. 2011;100(1):10–21.

Shander A, Goodnough LT. From tolerating anemia to treating anemia. Ann Intern Med. 2019;170(2):125–6.

Shander A, Gross I, Hill S, Javidroozi M, Sledge S. A new perspective on best transfusion practices. Blood Transfus. 2013;11(2):193.

Sharma AD, Sreeram G, Erb T, Grocott HP. Solvent-detergent–treated fresh frozen plasma: a superior alternative to standard fresh frozen plasma? J Cardiothorac Vasc Anesth. 2000;14(6):712–7.

Slichter SJ. Evidence-based platelet transfusion guidelines. Hematology. 2007;2007(1):172–8.

Strauss RG. Pretransfusion trigger platelet counts and dose for prophylactic platelet transfusions. Curr Opin Hematol. 2005;12(6):499–502.

Triulzi D, Aysola A, editors. Blood transfusion therapy: a physician's handbook. Bethesda, MD: AABB; 2002.

Wang JK, Klein HG. Red blood cell transfusion in the treatment and management of anaemia: the search for the elusive transfusion trigger. Vox Sang. 2010;98(1):2–11.

Whitaker BI, Hinkins S. The 2011 National Blood Collection and Utilization Survey report. Washington, DC: US Department of Health and Human Services; 2013.

Zielinski MD, Park MS, Jenkins D. Appropriate evidence-based practice guidelines for plasma transfusion would include a high ratio of plasma to red blood cells based on the available data. Transfusion. 2010;50(12):2762.

Zubair AC. Clinical impact of blood storage lesions. Am J Hematol. 2010;85(2):117–22.

5 Transfusion of blood & Its components

5.1 Introduction

Transfusion of whole blood and its components is frequent in the therapeutic medicine is used globally, and it is safe. Variation in red blood cell (RBC) transfusions persists across providers and is thought, in part, to be attributed to a lack of consensus regarding thresholds to support transfusion decision-making.

The subject of indication and contraindication of whole blood or its components depends on the following due to improved safety of blood transfusion (Box 5.1).

5.1.1 Reasons for Blood Transfusion

There is no simple laboratory or clinical indicators that determine the necessity for blood transfusion.

Box 5.1: Indication of Whole Blood and Its Components

To whom to give
What to give
When to give
How much to give
How to give

5.1.2 Oxygen Delivery

As the consideration of transfusion includes the combination of oxygen carrying and delivery, it should be noted that oxygen delivery is primarily determined by:

- Cardiac output
- Hemoglobin concentration
- Hemoglobin oxygen saturation

Final oxygen delivery is further dependent on the following:

- The oxygen diffusion gradient (determined in part by the hemoglobin oxygen affinity)
- The diffusion distance between the capillary and the cell
- Cellular uptake mechanisms

The theoretical critical hemoglobin (Hb) or hematocrit (Hct) threshold level required to maintain tissue oxygenation will vary dependent on the form of hypoxemia.

Transfusion of packed red blood cells (RBCs) provides three beneficial effects: circulatory (volume-related), rheological (viscosity-related), and oxygen carriage. Whole blood transfusion is currently restricted for volume expansion in cases of severe hemorrhage and

P. S. Ajmani, *Immunohematology and Blood banking*, https://doi.org/10.1007/978-981-15-8435-0_5

to increase viscosity only in cases of severe hemodilution. High viscosity in itself may impede circulation. Transfusion of specific blood components (pRBCS) is indicated to increase in oxygen delivery or utilization at the tissue level.

5.2 Transfusion Trigger

Transfusion trigger is defined as the value of hemoglobin (Hb) below which pRBC transfusion is indicated.

Transfusion target is the Hb one aims to achieve after RBC transfusion. Traditionally, the rule of "10/30" was followed for RBC transfusion, according to which Hb level of 10 g/dL or a hematocrit of 30% was recommended. Over the years, the trigger for transfusion has become more conservative or restrictive due to better options to treat anemia with specific medications. The decision to transfuse RBCs is based on the objective evaluation of the patient's clinical condition and her ability to compensate for the blood loss and its correlation with laboratory results. Therefore, the patient's age, severity of illness, comorbidities, and the rate and amount of hemorrhage are taken into account before transfusion (Table 5.1).

5.2.1 Transfusion Triggers

- **Perioperative transfusion**: 8 g/dL for patient undergoing cardiovascular surgery, acute GI bleeding, and major orthopedic surgeries like major joint replacements
  - Chronic anemia: –7 g/dL in adults
  - Acute blood loss: –30% of volume of blood
- **Transfusion yield**: One unit of whole blood/ pRBC can increase Hb by 1 g/dL in an adult or Hct by 3% (Hb of unit must be >75%) (Table 5.2).

5.3 Use of Blood Components

Whole blood: 450 mL whole blood in 63 mL anticoagulant-preservative solution of which Hb will be approximately 1.2 g/dL and hematocrit (Hct) 35–45% with no functional platelets or labile coagulation factors (V and VIII) when stored at +2 to +6 °C. Stored blood less than 7 days old is termed "fresh blood."

The indications of whole blood are limited to uncontrolled massive hemorrhage as occurs in victim of accidents and battle field injury and trauma patients, with a symptomatic deficit in oxygen-carrying capacity combined with hypovolemia of sufficient degree to be associated with shock.

Table 5.1 Showing blood components available for transfusion

Component	Composition	Volume (mL)
Whole blood	RBc + WBC + platelets	500
pRBC	RBC 75% + WBC + platelets + reduced plasma	250
pRBC + additive solution	pRBC 60% + WBC + platelets + reduced plasma + 100 mL of additive solution	330
leukocyte reduced pRBC	pRBCS >85%, few platelets + minimal plasma + <WBC 5×10^8	225
Washed RBCs	RBC >75% + WBC 5×10^8, no plasma	180
Frozen/deglycerolized RBC	RBC >75% + no platelets + no plasma + WBC <5×10^6	180
Platelet concentrate random donor	Platelets 5.5×10^6 + few RBC + WBC + plasma	50
Apheresis platelet	Platelet >3×10^{11}/unit + WBC <5×10^6 + plasma + minimum pRBCS	300
Apheresis granulocyte	Granulocyte >1×10^{10} + lymphocyte + some RBCs and platelets	220
Fresh frozen plasma	Plasma + all coagulation factors	220
Plasma	Plasma, stable clotting factors + no platelets	220
Cryoprecipitate	Factor VIII + von Willebrand + XIII + fibrinogen	15

Table 5.2 Showing clinical indication of blood components for transfusion

Blood components	Quantity	Clinical conditions
Whole blood	350–450 mL	Hypovolemia
pRBCs	150 –180 mL	Anemia
Fresh frozen plasma	140–180 mL	Bleeding disorders
Platelets	5×10^{10}	Platelet deficiency
Cryoprecipitate	80–100 units factor VIII	Factor VIII deficiency

Exchange transfusion in infants following hemolytic disease of the newborn.

All major surgery in infants and children.

In patients with extensive burn having increased plasma potassium level.

In cases of intravascular hemolysis: in neonate requiring exchange transfusion.

Only whole blood stored for less than 24 h at 20–24 °C can be considered a clinical source of viable platelets or therapeutic levels of labile coagulation factors V and VIII. Volume of blood required depends upon the patient's clinical condition, estimated loss of blood volume, and other measures being used to maintain hemodynamic stability.

Contraindications of whole blood: To avoid the risk of volume overload in patients with:

- Chronic anemia
- Incipient cardiac failure

If other effective measures to treat anemia are available such as iron, folic acid, vitamin B-12, and recombinant erythropoietin and when the patient's clinical condition permits sufficient time for these medications to promote erythropoiesis.

To increase blood volume when it can be safely and adequately replaced with volume expanders like normal saline, Hartmann's solution or appropriate colloids.

To correct coagulation disorder when they can be better treated with FFP and appropriate components and derivatives.

If a symptomatic deficiency in oxygen-carrying capacity can be better treated with packed red cell concentrate.

Infection risk: Capable of transmitting an infection present in cells or plasma which was undetected during routine screening for transfusion-transmitted infections like hepatitis B, hepatitis C, HIV 1 and 2, syphilis, and malaria.

5.4 Packed Red Blood Cells (pRBC)

Each unit of RCC contains 150–200 mL of red blood cells, from which most of the plasma has been removed. Hb concentration of the RCC will be approximately 20 g/100 mL (not less than 45 g per unit) and Hct 55–75%.

5.4.1 Indications of Packed Red Cells (pRBC)

Red cells are the primary cellular component used for the transfusion therapy in order to achieve a rapid increase in the supply of oxygen to the tissues, due to low hemoglobin and packed cell volume and/or the oxygen carrying capacity is reduced, in the presence of inadequate physiological mechanisms of compensation. When red cells are separated from the liquid plasma and used for transfusion, they are called packed red cells or red cell concentrate. Packed red cells are obtained by centrifugation of whole blood. Plasma is removed, and the resulting red cell suspension is transfused to the patient after diluting with sterile saline. Transfusion of packed red cells is reflected by the increase in hemoglobin and hematocrit value. Transfusion of red blood cells should be based on the patient's clinical condition (Box 5.2).

Box 5.2: Showing Indications for Transfusion of PRBCs

Anemia with clinical symptoms
Acute sickle cell crisis
Acute blood loss of more than 30% of blood volume

The signs of symptomatic anemia are shortness of breath, dizziness, congestive heart failure, and decreased exercise tolerance.

Box 5.3: Showing Types of Apheretic Red Cell Concentrate Available for Treatment of Anemia

RBC concentrates deprived of buffy coat
RBC concentrates with additive solutions (anticoagulants)
RBC concentrates deprived of the buffy coat and resuspended in additive solutions
Washed RBC
Leukodepleted RBC
Frozen RBC
Irradiated RBC

5.4.2 Life Span of Transfused Packed Red Blood Cell (Red Cell Concentrate)

The normal daily production of red blood cells (RBC) in a healthy adult is about 0.25 mL/kg, and the average lifespan of the cells is about 120 days, whereas that of transfused RBCs is about 50–60 days and can be significantly shorter in the presence of number of other factors reducing their survival (Boxes 5.3 and 5.4).

- **Infecstion risk**: It is same as for whole blood.
- **Storage**: It is same as for whole blood.

Box 5.4: Showing Inappropriate Indications for the Use of Packed Red Blood Cell

To increase blood volume
To replace iron, vit B-12 therapy, and folates
To accelerate wound healing
Anemia with Hb >10 g %
Monitoring indices for clinical auditing

5.4.3 Transfusion of pRBC or Red Cell Concentrates in Acute Anemia

The level of anemia that is tolerated without symptoms depends upon the patient's comorbidities and the degree of rapidity that the anemia develops.

Most patients will not require transfusions because they will have accommodated to the slowly developing anemia.

The decision to transfuse RBCs is based on hemoglobin concentration, PCV, the volume of blood loss, and the clinical condition of the patient.

The main therapeutic aim in the treatment of acute hemorrhage is to prevent or correct hypovolemic shock. In order to ensure tissue oxygenation, it is essential to restore circulatory volume by infusing crystalloids and colloids in sufficient amounts to maintain a satisfactory blood flow and blood pressure, before red cell concentrate is available.

A loss of less than 15% of the blood volume does not normally produce symptoms nor does it require transfusion, unless there is pre-existing anemia.

When the loss of volume is between 15% and 30%, a compensatory tachycardia develops, and the transfusion of pRBCs is indicated only in the presence of pre-existing anemia or concomitant cardiac or pulmonary disease.

Loss of blood due to any etiology and blood exceeding 30% of its volume can cause shock and require pRBC transfusion.

Blood loss of more than 40% results in development of severe shock, and then **transfusion becomes a life-saving intervention.**

Patients with Hb concentrations below 6 g/dL almost always require transfusion of packed red blood cells. In clinically stable patients with Hb level between 6 and 10 g/dL, the decision whether to transfuse is based on clinical status and laboratory results; patients with values above 10 g/dL rarely require transfusion.

5.4.3.1 False High Htc in Cases of Acute Hemorrhage

It is important to remember that patients with acute hemorrhage can have normal, or even high, PCV values until the plasma volume is restored; the clinical evaluation of the patient in this situation is therefore extremely important.

In cases of chronic anemia, 2,3-DPG level is increased in red blood cells, with a shift towards the right in the Hb dissociation curve and in the cardiac output and respiratory rate. For these reasons, pRBCs is rarely indicated in patients with Hb values above 8 g/dL.

5.4.4 Transfusion of pRBCs in Chronic Anemia

- **Hemoglobin <8 g %**: Find out the causes of anemia, and manage with other alternative. The use of hematinics in appropriate cases and erythropoietin in chronic renal failure or myelodysplastic syndromes is indicated.
- **Hemoglobin 8–10 g %**: Transfused pRBC is indicated when there is a marked decrease in oxygenation (abnormal cardio-circulatory or respiratory function).
- Patients receiving chemo therapeutic drugs and radiation therapy and in thrombocytopenic patients.
- **Hemoglobin 9–10 g %**: Patients with thalassemia.

5.4.4.1 Standard Transfusion Regimen for Thalassemia Major

Regular blood transfusions arise once in every 2–5 weeks to maintain the Hb >9–10.50.

5.4.4.2 Benefits

It allows normal physical activities and promotes normal growth in thalassemic patient.

It adequately suppresses bone marrow activity in most patients.

Hemoglobin level of >11–12 g/dL may be needed for patients with heart disease or other medical conditions for those patients who do not achieve adequate suppression of bone marrow activity at the lower Hb level.

5.4.4.3 Transfusion in Thalassemia

In this condition the threshold value is below 8–9 g/dL of Hb, in order to make a balance between inhibition of bone marrow erythropoiesis and iron overload which may develop after repeated transfusion therapy with pRBCs.

5.4.4.4 When to Start Transfusion in Thalassemia Major

Should be started after a definitive diagnosis by molecular study, Hb level, and PCV value, repeated on different occasions.

After confirmation of ineffective erythropoiesis by laboratory test and clinical criteria such as failure to thrive.

Positive radiological changes in bones.

The need for regular packed red cell transfusion for severe thalassemia usually occurs in the first 2 years of life.

Some patients with mild form of thalassemia who initially need occasional transfusions in the first two decades of life may later need regular transfusions because of a decreasing hemoglobin level, PCV, or the development of serious complications.

In patients with cardiac failure or very low initial hemoglobin levels, a smaller amount of packed red cells at slower rates of infusion is required.

Regular determinations of patient hemoglobin and packed cell volume allow assessment of the rate of fall in Hb level between transfusions and may be useful in evaluating the effects of changes in the transfusion regimen, the degree of hypersplenism, or unexplained changes in response to transfusion.

5.4.4.5 Packed RBC Indication in Sickle Cell Disease

In sickle cell disease, the fundamental indications for transfusion therapy with RBC are vascular occlusion and anemia.

Transfusion therapy is usually required in patients with Hb values <7 g/dL. In the presence of vascular occlusion, the aim of transfusion therapy is to prevent or stop intravascular sickling by dilution or replacement of the pathological circulating RBCs with normal RBCs; sickle cell patients must be transfused with pRBCs lacking Hb..

5.4.4.6 Packed RBC Indication in Patients Undergoing Chemotherapy

Patients undergoing chemotherapy or radiation therapy, who cannot wait for the effect of treatment with erythropoietin or in whom this hormone cannot be used because of specific receptors for it on the malignant cells, a suggested transfusion trigger for haemoglobin level of Hb concentration of 10 g/dL and PCV of 30 to counteract the protective effect of hypoxia on the neoplasia and to improve the pharmacokinetics of some chemotherapeutic agents in conditions of anemia.

5.4.4.7 Packed RBC Indications in Thrombocytopenia

The aim is to achieve the hemoglobin value of >10 g % and to reduce the risk of hemorrhage.

5.4.4.8 Packed RBC Transfusion in Surgery

Patients in clinically stable conditions and with Hb values ≥10 g/dL rarely require perioperative transfusions, while patients with Hb levels around 8 g/dL often require transfusion. Need for pRBC depends upon types of surgery, major or minor, the extent and speed of blood loss, and the presence of concomitant clinical conditions (age of the patient, heart and respiratory disorders).

Indication for autotransfusion: In cases of elective surgery for which the predicted transfusion requirements are at least 2 units of pRBCs and for which there is enough time to collect the autologous units and allow hematopoietic recovery.

5.4.5 Transfusion of pRBC in Bone Marrow Transplantation

The transfusion need for pRBC in bone marrow transplantation (BMT) varies greatly from patient to patient. All patients who are candidates for BMT require leukocyte-depleted red cells that are preferably of the same group and phenotype.

5.4.5.1 Percentage of Leucocytes Reduced by Blood Filters

Blood components filtered with the latest generation filters, able to reduce the leukocyte content by 99.9%, are a valid alternative to cytomegalovirus (CMV)-negative blood components.

Transfusion in allogenic bone marrow transplant should be transfused with irradiated blood components until the start of their conditioning chemotherapy or radiotherapy. This indication also continues until **graft-versus-**host disease (GvHD) prophylaxis is given: usually for 6 months or until the lymphocyte count exceeds 1000/μL.

Packed red blood cell indications in patients transplanted for combined immunodeficiency diseases or with chronic GvHD require irradiated blood components for a longer period of more than 2 years.

Aim for transfusion in transplanted patients: The aim of transfusion during the phase of thrombocytopenia is to maintain the hemoglobin value of more than 10 g % and packed cell volume of more than 30 to reduce the risk of hemorrhage.

The ABO and Rh (D) group of pRBCs to be transfused during allogeneic BMT must be contemporaneously compatible with the donor's and recipient's group.

Frozen red blood cells must be stored at −65 °C and should be transfused within 10 years.

Transfusion of packed red blood cell (red cell concentrate (RCC)) in neonates: Neonates require smaller volume (25–100 mL) which can be prepared by fractionating a standard unit of pRBC into several aliquots; these aliquots can be transfused in succession, in this way reducing the number of donors to which the recipient is exposed.

Packed RBC used in the neonatal transfusion must be leukodepleted, preferably at the time of collection (prestorage), but at any rate, within 72 h of collection.

In order to prevent GvHD, pRBC must be irradiated when used in the situations listed in the paragraph concerning irradiated pRBC.

The threshold value of Hb in the neonate (10 g/dL) is higher than that in the adult and even higher (12–13 g/dL) in the first 24 h of life or in the presence of cardiac or respiratory failure.

5.4.5.2 Dose of pRBC

The generally recommended doses of pRBC are 5–20 mL/kg.

Patients suffering from chronic anemia resulting due to renal failure or gastrointestinal bleeding responded well.

5.4.5.3 Indications for Leukodepleted pRBC

The presence of leukocytes in a unit of pRBC can fragment, deteriorate, and release cytokines and causes reactions to current and subsequent blood transfusions in some patients.

- Prevention of the transmission of CMV in CMV-negative patients with congenital or acquired immunodeficiency
- CMV-negative recipients of a BMT from a CMV-negative donor
- Patients who need prolonged transfusion support
- Prevention of recurrent febrile non-hemolytic transfusion reactions
- Prevention of refractoriness to platelet transfusion
- In pregnant women, independent of their CMV serological status, in order to avoid the possible immunomodulatory effect of the transfusion (reactivation of CMV)

Renal transplantation: The use of leukodepleted red cells prevents HLA alloimmunization and avoids the risk of transmission of CMV.

Immunomodulation: There is not sufficient evidence to recommend routine use of leukodepleted RBCs in surgical patients, with the aim of preventing post-operative infections or recurrent neoplastic changes.

- To reduce the risk of rejection in patients for hematopoietic stem cell transplantation
- Intrauterine transfusions
- Transfusions in premature or low-birth-weight babies
- Transfusion in neonate's up to 1 year of age

Gamma irradiation of whole blood, red cell, and apheresis platelet units with 25–50 Gy renders lymphocytes incapable of proliferation Irradiation and is currently the only method available for preventing transfusion-related GvHD.

5.4.6 Indications of Irradiated pRBC

ALL designated donotions.

Blood components selected based on HLA compatibility.

Intrauterine transfusion and subsequent transfusion in neonates with a birth weight of ≤1500 g and/or gestational age ≤30 weeks.

Newborns with erythroblastosis fetalis.

Patients with congenital cellular immunodeficiency.

Patients with **Hodgkin's disease**, neuroblastoma, and sarcoma.

Patients receiving purine analogs (e.g., fludarabine).

Peripheral blood stem cell or marrow transplant.

Prevention of alloimmunization to donor HLA antigens (i.e., platelet-dependent patients who may become refractory to platelet transfusions; leukoreduced RBCs still contain enough leukocytes capable of producing transfusion-associated graft-versus-host disease (*TAGVHD*) in susceptible patients). Prevention of TAGVHD can only be accomplished by irradiation of the RBC unit.

Patients undergoing chemotherapy should be decided on the basis of immunosuppression.

Transfusion with blood components donated by first- or second-degree relatives (excluding stem cells and lymphocyte concentrates).

Allogeneic transplant (until the end of GvHD prophylaxis or a lymphocyte count $>1 \times 10^9$/L is reached).

Bone marrow donation for allogeneic transplantation (allogeneic blood components transfused to the donor before and during explantation).

Bone marrow or peripheral blood stem cell (PBSC) autologous transplantation (in the 7 days before collection of bone marrow or PBSC and up to 3 months after transplantation or 6 months for patients undergoing total body irradiation).

When none of the above conditions are present, it is not necessary to irradiate blood components transfused to patients with HIV infection or aplastic anemia and patients undergoing solid organ transplantation and chemotherapy for non-Hodgkin's lymphoma, acute leukemias, and solid tumors.

HIV infection is not an indication for irradiated blood product.

5.4.6.1 Side Effect of Irradiated pRBC

The irradiated pRBC results in increased potassium level which is due to the accelerated release of potassium from the erythrocytes which can cause serious problems in the case of intrauterine transfusions or exchange transfusions.

5.4.7 Indications of Washed pRBC

Recurrent febrile non-hemolytic transfusion reactions (RFNTR) not prevented by leukocyte reduction and antipyretics.

Recurrent severe allergic transfusion reactions such as urticarial reactions not prevented by pre-transfusion antihistamine and corticosteroid administration.

History of severe anaphylactoid reaction with previous transfusion.

To prevent anaphylactic transfusion reactions in IgA deficiency patients with documented anti-IgA antibodies.

Depletion of potassium and anticoagulants prior to transfusion to a fetus or to a neonate with renal failure or when large amount of RBC component is needed for neonate (i.e., RBC exchange, dialysis, extracorporeal membrane oxygenation (ECMO)) when fresh RBCs are not available. Maternal platelets collected for neonates with neonatal alloimmune thrombocytopenia (controversial). Atypical HUS with T-antigen activation (controversial).

Washed RBC unit may increase Hb content by 70% only because 10–20% of the RBCs are lost in the washing process; in addition there is 33% loss of platelet product during the washing process. The platelet's functionality may also be altered providing a suboptimal response.

Indications of frozen red cells: Patients with complex immunohematological profiles when compatible donors are not available.

Use frozen red cells for red cells with unusual phenotypes and for autologous collections when liquid-preserved blood cannot fulfill demands. These are for patients with rare red cell phenotypes or multiple red cell antibodies.

Autologous collection of blood for potential future use.

Quarantined allogeneic O-positive and O-negative red cells can be frozen for greater than 6 months, during which time the donor can be retested for infectious disease markers.

Rare type and selected red cells can be saved.

Red cells with improved oxygen transport function are especially useful in coronary artery and cerebrovascular disease, cardiopulmonary bypass surgery, and hypothermia.

Patients with immunoglobulin A (IgA) deficiency.

In paroxysmal nocturnal hemoglobinuria (PNH).

Rare and autologous red cells can be refrozen after thawing.

Red blood cells (RBCs) can be cryopreserved with shelf life of 10 years. However, shelf life of deglycerolized RBCs in conventional open system is just 24 h, resulting in sporadic use of frozen RBC (FS-RBC). It is essential to remove the glycerol from thawed component prior to transfusion. This is done by washing the cells with normal saline. The washed red cells are then resuspended in additive solution.

The most important of these uses is the quarantine of allogeneic frozen red cells, i.e., the use of freeze-preservation as a means of avoiding the potential for transmission of disease through an allogeneic transfusion. It is now possible to quarantine frozen donor red blood cells for at least 6 months to retest the donor for pathogens that were undetectable at donation.

5.4.8 Adverse Reactions of Packed Red Blood Cell

Transfusion therapy with pRBCs can cause adverse reactions, which are classified into four categories on the basis of their etiopathogenesis and the time of occurrence with respect to the transfusion.

5.5 Fresh Frozen Plasma (FFP)

Fresh frozen plasma (FFP) is the liquid portion of blood that is prepared either from the primary centrifugation of whole blood into red cells and plasma or from a secondary centrifugation of platelet-rich plasma and frozen at −30 °C or colder within 8 h of whole blood donation if the anticoagulant used was CPD, CD2D, or CPDA-1 and within 6 h if the anticoagulant was ACD. FFP contains all the coagulation factors, including fibrinogen and factor VIII.

FFP is thawed before transfusion 30–37 °C in water bath for 20–30 min.

There is no lower temperature limit for the storage of FFP.

5.5.1 Indications for Fresh Frozen Plasma (FFP)

Replacement of a single coagulation factor deficiency, in absence of a specific or combined factor deficiency.

Reversal of warfarin effect, when prothrombin complex concentrate is not available.

Thrombotic thrombocytopenic purpura.

Inherited coagulation inhibitor deficiencies where specific concentrate is unavailable.

C1 esterase inhibitor deficiency where specific concentrate is unavailable.

5.5.2 Conditional Indications for Fresh Frozen Plasma (FFP)

Massive blood transfusion.

Acute DIC if there are coagulation abnormalities in bleeding patient.

Liver diseases with abnormal coagulation and bleeding time.

Prophylactic use to have normal prothrombin time in case of liver biopsy.

Cardiopulmonary bypass surgery: use in the presence of bleeding but where abnormal coagulation is not due to heparin. Routine perioperative use is not indicated.

Neonatal septicemia (independent of DIC).

Plasmapheresis.

5.5.3 Difference Between Fresh Frozen Plasma and Plasma Frozen

FFP must be made and frozen within 8 h of collection, where as plasma frozen within 24 h after phlebotomy is prepared and then frozen.

FFP contains some what higher levels of factor V and VIII, but the levels in plasma frozen within 24 h after phlebotomy are comparatively less (Box 5.5).

Box 5.5: Showing Different Types of Plasma

Fresh frozen plasma (FFP)
p24 plasma
Plasma
Thawed plasma
Cryoreduced plasma
Source plasma
Recovered plasma
Donor retested plasma
Methylene blue treated FFP (MBFFP)
Solvent-detergent treated plasma (SDFFP)
Jumbo fresh frozen plasma
PF24 PF24RT24

p24 plasma is the same as FFP except that the separation and centrifugation occurred between 8 and 24 h of collection. P24 plasma therefore may have decreased amounts of labile proteins such as factors VIII (8) and V (5).

Plasma: Plasma removed from liquid whole blood between 24 h after collection and up to 5 days after the expiration of the whole blood unit product is stored and frozen at ≤−65 up to 7 years.

Thawed plasma is defined as previously frozen plasma in the blood bank at 1–6 °C that has been thawed and issued up to 5 days after thawing. Whole blood derived FFP or FP24 product as "thawed plasma" and keep at the same storage conditions for up to 5 days from the time of thawing.

Thawed plasma is considered by most to be functionally equivalent to thawed FFP and is used interchangeably in most clinical situations. The characteristics of thawed plasma are the following:

- Moderate decreases in both factor V and factor VIII are seen.
- Roughly half the levels present at the time of thawing are seen at the 5-day expiration time.
- However, this is not seen as an impediment to the use of the product, as factors remain in the range that can still induce hemostasis.
- It is not good for factor VIII replacement.
- When available, thawed plasma will be issued for the same indications as FFP. The level of stable clotting factors remains the same as in FFP, and labile factors V and VIII remain at 75–95% (FV) and 45–75% (FVIII) levels, respectively. Thawed plasma should not be used as sole source for f actor VIII replacement, and factor VIII concentrate is a better option.

Cryoreduced plasma (CRP): In order to produce cryoprecipitate (Cryo, antihemophilic factor/AHF), FFP is thawed at 1–6 °C, and a small amount of solid material (precipitate) is left behind. The fluid that is removed (15 mL) is called "cryoreduced plasma," also known as "cryo-poor plasma" and "cryosupernatant." FFP-CRP contains decreased levels of the components of Cryo (fibrinogen, factors VIII and XIII, and von Willebrand factor) but near-normal levels of the rest of the coagulation factors. CRP really has main indication for transfusion or fluid replacement in cases of thrombotic thrombocytopenic purpura. Storage times and temperature of CRP are identical to those for FFP.

Source plasma definition: This product is not available in the blood bank but is sourced from pharmacy. It has the following characteristics:

- Product collected by apheresis, from paid donors.
- Intended for manufacture into either injectable or non-inject able products.
- Donors are subjected for same infectious diseases as regular blood donors.
- Licensed product collected only by licensed facilities.

5.5.4 Recovered Plasma Characteristics

Plasma separated from volunteer whole blood donation (in contrast to source plasma).

Unlicensed product.

Unused units of FFP, FP24, or plasma may be re-labeled as recovered plasma at any time.

Blood bank may use recover plasma as source of revenue, selling product for further manufacture through "short supply agreements" with plasma companies.

5.5.5 Donor-Retested Plasma

It is another uncommonly used plasma product.

The donor blood should be screened twice for infectious disease by two different kits before his plasma is released for transfusion.

The unit of plasma is held until the donor has been re-tested at a regular donation interval (at least 56 days); if negative, first unit is released.

Pathogen-reduced plasma components are of two types; they are:

Methylene blue treated FFP (MBFFP)
Solvent-detergent treated plasma (SDFFP)

Methylene blue treated FFP (MBFFP) is leukocyte-depleted plasma that has been obtained from whole blood or by apheresis from a previously tested donor, contains less than 1×10^6 leucocytes, and has been treated with methylene blue and exposed to visible light to inactivate pathogens. The MBT contains methylene blue concentration ≤0.30 μmol/L (less than approximately 30 μg per unit).

The **MBT process** reduces the FVIII: C content by approximately 30% when compared to standard fresh frozen plasma.

Intact white blood cells in the plasma should be reduced to less than 1×10^6 per unit prior to exposure to methylene blue and visible light.

The solvent-detergent treated plasma (SDFFP): Aim is to inactivate enveloped viruses in plasma protein preparation. The method proved effective in the processing of coagulation factor concentrates by disrupting the membranes of lipid-enveloped viruses, cells, and most protozoa while leaving the labile coagulation factors intact. Its efficacy to inactivate bacteria is variable, and it is ineffective against non-lipid-enveloped viruses. SD appears to be associated with a lower risk of transfusion-related acute lung injury (TRALI) and allergic reactions. The SD treatment of plasma results in a prompt and large reduction of enveloped viruses. SD treatment has no effect on non-enveloped viruses (Box 5.6). **The enveloped viruses of importance in transfusion which can be inactivated are as under.**

Box 5.6: Showing List of Enveloped Viruses

HBV
HCV
HIV 1 and 2
HAV (hepatitis A virus)
Parvo virus B 19

5.5.6 Jumbo Fresh Frozen Plasma (Jumbo FFP)

A unit of jumbo FFP is equivalent to 2 units of FFP because it is collected by an apheresis machine.

5.5.7 Fresh Frozen Plasma (FFP), PF24, PF24RT24, and Cryoreduced Plasma

When one of the above products is thawed for transfusion, it must be stored in the refrigerator (1–6 °C) if not transfused immediately. The product technically has only a 24-h shelf life, but the "Circular of Information" describes a pathway to avoid discarding an unused product at the end of the 24 h. The products above may be relabeled as "Thawed Plasma" (note the CAPITAL "T" and "P") and stored under the same conditions as before (i.e., 1–6 °C) for up to 5 days after thawing (technically, cryoreduced plasma must be relabeled as "Thawed Plasma Cryoprecipitate Reduced," but the principle is the same). Most facilities use Thawed Plasma for exactly the same indications as the original component, with the possible exception that, due to the documented decrease in factor VIII and to a lesser extent factors V and protein S, some will limit its use in cases of consumptive coagulopathies like DIC.

Table 5.3 Showing properties of different types of plasma

Properties	SD	MB	FFP	Intercept	Mirasol
Pathogen inactivation	Yes	Yes	No	Yes	Yes
Free of cells and cell fragments	Yes	No	No	No	No
No risk of TRALI	Yes	No	No	No	No
Reduced allergic reactions	Yes	No	No	No	No
Coagulation factor potencies	Yes	No	No	No	No
Clinical efficacy	Yes	No	Yes	Yes	?

FFP fresh frozen plasma, *MB* methylene blue, *SD* solvent/detergent, *TRALI* transfusion-related acute lung insufficiency

5.5.7.1 PF24RT24

PF24RT24 stands for "Plasma frozen within 24 h after phlebotomy held at room temperature for up to 24 h, PF24RT24 can **stay at room temperature for the entire time** between collection and freezer placement." This product has decreased factor V and factor VIII when compared to FFP (though, like PF24, the decrease in factor VIII is more pronounced than the decrease in factor V (13% decreased for FVIII vs. 1% for factor V). The coagulation inhibitor protein S is also decreased by about 10% in PF24RT24 when compared to FFP. A couple of facts are pertinent about this product: Unlike PF24, which can come from an apheresis or whole blood collection, this product is only approved for apheresis collections. Individual apheresis-derived plasma units may be larger than units of either FFP or PF24. Second, like PF24, it can be kept for up to 5 days after thawing (it can be relabeled as "Thawed Plasma" after the first 24 h of storage). Finally, like PF24, it **can't be** used to make cryoprecipitate (due to decreased levels of FVIII). For comparison, here are the three products compared in terms of processing.

5.5.8 Processing Terms

5.5.8.1 FFP

- In freezer (at <−30 °C) within 8 h of collection

5.5.8.2 PF24

- In refrigerator (at 1–6 °C) within 8 h of collection
- In freezer (at <−30 °C) within 24 h of collection

5.5.8.3 PF24RT24

- Room temperature (20–24 °C) for up to 24 h after collection
- In freezer (at <−30 °C) within 24 h of collection (Table 5.3)

5.5.9 Intercept Blood System for Plasma

The **intercept** blood system is intended to inactivate a broad spectrum of viruses, bacteria, and parasite as well as contaminating donor leukocytes in platelet components.

Intercept treatment may be used in place of cytomegalovirus (CMV) testing and leukoreduction for prevention of transfusion-transmitted CMV infection.

The Mirasol PRT system reduces the pathogen load of a broad range of disease-causing viruses, bacteria, and parasites in blood components including platelets. The system also inacti-

Box 5.7: Showing Contents of Fresh Frozen Plasma

Clotting factors
Fibrinogen
Prothrombin
Globulin
Albumin

vates residual white blood cells found in blood components, which may help to reduce transfusion reactions in patients. The method is very effective in "window period" (Box 5.7).

Storage temperature of fresh frozen plasma (FFP) and cryoprecipitate: FFP bags should be frozen in a horizontal position and stored at vertical position (Table 5.4).

Unit of issue: One unit contains 200–250 mL of anticoagulated plasma with approximately 400–500 mg of fibrinogen. Each mL of plasma contains 0.7–1.0 activity unit of all other clotting factors.

Dosage and timings: 15 mL/kg. Administration: Should be ABO compatible.

Before transfusion FFP has to be thaw; it will take 30 min.

Labile coagulation factors rapidly degrade; use within 6 h of thawing.

FFP should be administered within 30 min after thawing but can be transfused up to 24 h provided it has been maintained at 1 –6 °C.

The infusion of FFP will be determined on the basis of laboratory findings. If the PT and PTT are within 1.5 times the normal limits (INR <1.5).

If PT and PTT test were not determined in the past 24 h.

5.5.9.1 Exceptions

Patients with PT and PTT 1.0–1.5 times normal and significant bleeding (≥4 units in 24 h).

Trauma or traumatic brain patients can receive FFP regardless of INR.

Table 5.4 Showing storage temperature of fresh frozen plasma (FFP) and cryoprecipitate

Product storage	Temperature	Maximum storage time
FFP	–65 °C or below	7 years
FFP or cryoprecipitate	–40 to –64 °C	24 months
FFP or cryoprecipitate	–30 to –39 °C	12 months
FFP or cryoprecipitate	–25 to –29 °C	6 months
FFP or cryoprecipitate	–20 to –24 °C	3 months
P24 plasma	–20 to –24 °C	3 months
Apheresis FFP	–20 to –24 °C	3 months
Liquid plasma	4 °C	5 days
Thawed plasma	4 °C	6 h
Cryoprecipitated AHF	–20 to –24 °C	3 months
Cryoprecipitated reduced plasma after thawing	4 °C	5 days

The dose of FFP used should be adequate for replacement of coagulation factors. For example, an adult with liver disease will usually require 3–9 units (10–15 mL/kg body weight) of FFP to clinically significantly shorten the PT.

FFP should be administered at the time of bleeding or within an hour of the anticipated bleeding. The maximal effect of FFP declines 2–4 h after transfusion.

For urgent reversal of warfarin anticoagulation, a lower FFP dose (5–8 mL/kg) may be sufficient although full correction to an INR of 1.5 or less will usually require the full adult dose. In life-threatening bleeding situations related to warfarin overdose, treatment with a prothrombin complex concentrate (available from pharmacy) should be considered. Intermediate purity pooled plasma products containing a mixture of vitamin K-dependent proteins.

5.5.10 Monitoring of Effective Treatment with FFP

Perform pretransfusion and post transfusion of PT and aPTT immediately after the transfusion of FFP.

Infection risk: Capable of transmitting any agent present in cells or plasma which was undetected by routine screening of transfusion-transmitted infection including HIV, hepatitis B and C, syphilis, and malaria (Box 5.8).

Precautions: Acute allergic reactions are not uncommon, especially with rapid infusions. Severe life-threatening anaphylactic reactions occasionally occur.

Plasma thawing equipment: This is a specially designed water bath able to maintain constant temperature at around +37 °C.

Defrosting FFP pack from −30 to 0 °C will take approximately 20 min.

Types of thawer: They are of two types, wet and dry thawers.

- **Wet thawer**: The plasma packs are suspended from clamps and packed to be in direct contact with the water; detergent should never be added to the water.
- **Dry thawer**: In this type of thawer, the plasma packs are protected from direct contact with the water by leak-proof containers (bladders) that come as part of the equipment. The warm water is circulated around the bags. The "dry" type of thawer is ideal because the operator's hands and the plasma packs remain dry.

Box 5.8: Showing Risks Associated with FFP

Hepatitis B and C
HIV 1 and 2
Minor allergic reactions like urticarial
Severe allergic reactions like bronchospasm and anaphylactic reaction
Fluid overload
Transfusion-related acute lung injury (TRALI)

Humate-P antihaemophilic factor also known as (Human Plasma-derived von Willebrand Factor) or (factor IX complex), Prothrombin complex (PCC): It contains both vWF and factor VIII.

Indications: It is very effective in hemophilia A (classical hemophilia) (can also use factor VIII); FFP does not work effectively.

Von Willebrand disease that is unresponsive to **desmopressin** (DDAVP) (can use cryoprecipitate); FFP does not work effectively.

In spontaneous or trauma-induced bleeding episodes in adults and children with von Willebrand disease (VWD) and prevents excessive bleeding during and after surgery in patients with mild, moderate, or severe VWD.

Contraindication: Hypersensitivity to Humate-P or its products.

Humate-P is made from human blood and could contain infectious agents. The risk that these agents may transmit disease cannot be completely eliminated but has been reduced by screening plasma donors and testing donated plasma (Boxes 5.9 and 5.10 and Table 5.5).

Dosing of PCC: Although questions persist regarding the minimum effective dose and the

Box 5.9: Showing Advantages of Prothrombin Complex Concentrate (PCC) in Relation to FFP

More effective and rapid correction of INR
Greater increase in clotting factors
Require less volume and can be administered faster than FFP
Less number of complications secondary to fluid overload
Shorter preparation time since PCC does not need to be thawed as FFP
Does not require blood type matching

Box 5.10: Showing Side Effect of Humate-P

Headache
Vomiting
Sleepiness
Pulmonary embolism
Blood clots
Deep vein thrombosis

Box 5.11: Showing Contents of Cryoprecipitate

von Willebrand's factor
Fibrinogen: 150–300 mg in each unit
Factor VIII: about 80 IU in each unit
Fibronectin

Table 5.5 Showing composition of prothrombin complex concentrate

Beriplex	FII	FVII	FIX[a]	FX	Dose
	128 units	68 units	100 units	152 units	25–50 units/kg

maximum safe dose, the average dose recommended for reversal of supratherapeutic INR is 25–50 units/kg, based upon the factor IX component. Each of the PCC formulations contains varying amounts of factors II, VII, IX, and X. Additionally, the amount of factor varies between vials of the same preparation.

Route of administration: Slow IV injection.

5.5.11 Cryoprecipitate

Cryoprecipitated antihemophilic factor (AHF) or "cryo" is prepared from FFP by collecting the precipitate formed during controlled thawing at +4 °C and resuspending in 10–20 mL plasma. It is stored at −30 °C or colder for up to 1 year after the date of phlebotomy (Box 5.11).

5.5.11.1 Indications for Cryoprecipitate

(a) **Hypofibrinogenemia or afibrinogenemia**, in association with bleeding or prior to an invasive procedure:

Hypofibrinogenemia may be due to:

Lack of synthesis (e.g., liver disease).

Consumption of coagulation factors in cases of massive hemorrhage like abruptio placentae, amniotic fluid embolism, disseminated intravascular coagulation [DIC], and treatment with asparaginase.

Dilution: in cases of massive blood transfusion (MBT) or intensive plasma exchange).

Inherited deficiency.

(b) **Any of the following conditions** in association with bleeding or prior to surgery:

1. **von Willebrand disease** when desmopressin (DDAVP) is ineffective or contraindicated and non-availability of von Willebrand factor.
2. **Dysfibrinogenemias**, both inherited and acquired (e.g., due to liver disease).
3. **Hemophilia A**: when factor VIII concentrate is not available and administration of DDAVP is not indicated.

(c) **Factor XIII deficiency** in association with bleeding. Cryoprecipitate may be indicated for replacement in the case of factor XIII deficiency.

FFP may also be used, but infusion requires much larger volumes.

Factor XIII concentrate has been used for prophylactic treatment of congenital factor XIII deficiency, but not for bleeding episodes.

In patients with uremia: If the bleeding is unresponsive to other treatment modalities, such as DDAVP, estrogen, red cell transfusions, dialysis, and erythropoietin.

Ameliorate platelet dysfunction associated with uremia.

Box 5.12: Showing Indications for Transfusion of Cryoprecipitate (Summary)

Thrombocytopenic purpura (TTP)
Treatment for factor VIII deficiency (hemophilia A)
Congenital or acquired fibrinogen deficiency
FXIII deficiency

Used topically as a fibrin sealant (Box 5.12).

Infection risk: As for plasma, but a normal adult dose involves at least 6 donor exposures.

5.5.11.2 Cryoprecipitate Administration

Cryoprecipitate needs not be ABO compatible, but ABO group compatibility is essential in infants and in children. Cryoprecipitates should be administered within 4 h of thawing; it will take 30 min. Cryoprecipitate is available in pool of 5.

Fibrinogen replacement requires 2 units of pooled cryoprecipitate/10 kg of body weight which will raise fibrinogen concentration by 100 mg/dL, except in cases of DIC or continued bleeding with massive transfusion. Therapy should be based on clinical status, with object of achieving and maintaining a fibrinogen concentration of 100 mg/dL, as clinically indicated.

Fibrinogen replacement: Effect can be monitored by clinical response to therapy and fibrinogen level assay.

5.5.11.3 Dosage

This product is available in pools of 5 units.

- One bag contains 80 units of factor VIII: C (AHF) and 325 mg fibrinogen
- Five bags (1 pool) contains 1625 mg fibrinogen
- Recovery rate with transfusion = 75%
- Five bags of cryoprecipitate provides 1220 mg fibrinogen
- 70 kg × 0.05 = plasma volume of 35 dL (3.5 L)
- 1220 mg = 35 mg/dL provided by 5 bag pool of cryoprecipitate

In a 70 kg patient: 5 bags (1 pool) of cryo raises fibrinogen 35 mg/dL.

Pediatric dosing for cyroprecipitate is 1 unit per 10 kg child, which should increase fibrinogen by 60–100 mg/dL.

Von Willebrand disease (vWD): Cryo should only be used in vWD patients who do not respond to DDAVP and when vWD-containing FVIII concentrate (Humate-P) is not available. The loading dose for cryo is calculated from the desired versus actual patient VIII: C activity as described below. Repeat dose every 12–24 h, monitoring F VIII: C levels.

To replace factor VIII or von Willebrand factor: When specific factor concentrates are unavailable, the usual adult dose is a pool of 5–10 bags. Approximately 150 units of factor VIII and von Willebrand factor are provided per bag. A single donor may be used repeatedly for a young or mildly affected patient to limit donor exposures.

5.5.11.4 Dose Calculation

If X% is the desired plasma F VIII: C level, the number of F VIII: C units to be given IV are X/2 per kg of body weight. Since the half-life of F VIII: C is approximately 12 h, the maintenance dose is 1/2 the initial dose given every 12 h. For example, to achieve 100% F VIII:C level in a 50 kg patient, (100/2) × 50 = 2500 units are given initially by IV, and 1250 units are given by IV every 12 h thereafter. These guidelines assume pretreatment F VIII: C levels of 0%.

Hemophilia A: Drug of choice in mild to moderate cases of hemophilia A is DDAVP and/or factor VIII concentrates. Cryo should only be used for hemophilia in cases when F VIII products are not available.

5.5.11.5 Suggested Target Levels for FVIII Replacement

Minor bleeding, for example, into the joints: 30% F VIII: C with or without maintenance therapy.

Major bleeding examples are intracranial, retroperitoneal, nervous system involvement, mouth or tongue, deep muscle, hematuria, major surgery – 100% F VIII: maintained between 50% and 100% for at least several days.

Hemophilia A: patients presenting with bleeding usually have F VIII: C levels near 0%.

Fibrinogen deficiency: For fibrinogen levels <100 mcg/dL and significant bleeding (or risk thereof), usual adult dose is 10 units of cryoprecipitate or two pools of 5. It will raise the fibrinogen level approximately 100 mcg/dL.

Bleeding Caused by the Use of Streptokinase or TPA.

Human Fibrin Glue (HFG) is the drug of choice in bleeding and commercially available in the market by the name of TISSEEL used for hemostasis: TISSEEL is a fibrin sealant indicated for use as an adjunct to hemostasis in adult and pediatric patients (>1 month of age) undergoing surgery when control of bleeding by conventional surgical techniques (such as suture, ligature, and cautery) is ineffective or impractical. TISSEEL is effective in heparinized patients.

TISSEEL consists of two components contained in separate vials: a freeze-dried concentrate of clotting proteins, mainly fibrinogen, factor XIII, and fibronectin (the sealant), and freeze-dried thrombin (the catalyst). These are loaded into two syringes with tips forming a common port. When injected the two components meet in equal volumes at the point of delivery. The thrombin converts the fibrinogen to fibrin by enzymatic action at a rate determined by the concentration of thrombin. The more concentrated thrombin solution produces a fibrin clot in about 10 s, and the more dilute thrombin solution forms the clot about 60 s after the glue is applied to the surgical field.

Currently, tissue glue is being used for amniotic membrane transplantation, conjunctival closure following pterygium and strabismus surgery, forniceal reconstruction surgery, lamellar corneal grafting, closure of corneal perforations and descematoceles, management of conjunctival wound leaks after trabeculectomy, lid surgery, and adnexal surgery and as a hemostat to minimize bleeding. It is also used in reconstructive and orthopedic procedures and to prevent leakage from colonic anastomoses following the reversal of temporary colostomies.

Risk factors: For topical use only. Do not inject TISSEEL directly into the circulatory system or into highly vascularized tissue. Intravascular application of TISSEEL can lead to intravascular coagulation, can result in life-threatening thromboembolic events, and can increase the likelihood and severity of acute hypersensitivity reactions in susceptible patients.

Do not use TISSEEL in individuals with a known hypersensitivity to aprotinin.

TISSEEL should be applied as a thin layer by dripping or spraying using cannula or spray set.

It is not indicated for the treatment of severe or brisk arterial or venous bleeding.

Desmopressin (DDAVP) is the drug of choice to treat hemophilia A and von Willebrand disease of mild to moderate cases. It may be given by oral route under the tongue, in the nose, or by IV. If desmopressin is not available, then patient should be given cryoprecipitate.

5.6 Platelets

Platelets are small, disc-shaped cells that have a critical role in maintaining hemostasis and helping our blood clot and stop bleeding. When there is a break in the vascular endothelium, a process of platelet activation occurs, and the platelets change shape and aggregates to form a platelet plug known as primary hemostatis.

Platelet concentrates (PC) are prepared from units of whole blood that have not been allowed to cool below +20 °C. A single donor unit consists of 50–60 mL plasma that should contain $\geq 55 \times 10^9$ platelets.

5.6.1 Indication of Platelet Transfusion

Platelet transfusion is usually required in a bleeding patient below a platelet count of 50×10^9/L but rarely above 100×10^9/L. If the values fall between these two, transfusion is considered in case of platelet dysfunction (e.g., clopidogrel therapy), ongoing bleeding, and surgeries in confined spaces such as eye and brain.

Indications: Treatment of bleeding due to:

- Thrombocytopenia
- Platelet function defects
- Prevention of bleeding due to thrombocytopenia as occurs in bone marrow failure

Prophylactic use: In thrombocytopenic patients.

Contraindications of platelet transfusion:

- Idiopathic autoimmune thrombocytopenic purpura (ITP)
- Thrombotic thrombocytopenic purpura (TTP)
- Untreated DIC thrombocytopenia associated with septicemia or in cases of hypersplenism

Goal of the treatment

- In non-bleeding, non-infected patient, maintain platelet count $>10 \times 10^9$/L.
- In infected patient and in patient with pyrexia, maintain platelet count $>20 \times 10^9$/L.
- In cases of acute DIC, where bleeding is associated with thrombocytopenia, maintain platelet count above 20×10^9/L, even in the absence of overt bleeding.

In massive blood transfusion (MBT), maintain platelet count $>50 \times 10^9$/L.

In MBT, dilutional thrombo cytopenia occurs when $>1.5 \times$ blood volume of patient is transfused.

Use in cardiopulmonary bypass surgery: thrombocytopenia and platelet function defects often occur after cardiac bypass surgery.

Platelet transfusion is recommended for patients with bleeding not due to surgically correctable causes (closure time provides global indication of platelet function).

Prophylactic platelet transfusions are not required for all bypass procedures.

Prophylaxis for surgery: Platelet count should be $>50 \times 10^9$/L for therapeutic and diagnostic procedures; if the count falls below the required value, prophylactic use of platelet infusion is indicated in conditions as under (Box 5.13).

Maintain platelet count $>100 \times 10^9$/L for neurological and ophthalmic surgery.

- **Administration**: Platelet concentrates after pooling should be infused with in 30 min, because of the risk of bacterial proliferation.
- **Complications**: Allergic urticarial reactions and febrile non-hemolytic are not uncommon, especially in patients receiving multiple transfusions.
- **Unit of issue**: PCs may be supplied as a pooled unit, i.e., platelets prepared from 4–6 donor units containing at least 240×10^9 platelets.
- **Infection risk**: Bacterial contamination affects about 1% of pooled units.

Box 5.13: Showing Indications for Prophylaxis Use of Platelets

Lumbar puncture
Insertion of indwelling lines
Transbronchial biopsy
Epidural anesthesia
Renal biopsy
Liver biopsy
Laparotomy

- **Storage**: PCs may be stored for up to 5 days at +20 to +24 °C (with agitation). PCs require continuous agitation during storage, on a platelet shaker and in an incubator that maintains the required storage temperature.
- **Dosage**: It depends upon the body weight: one unit of platelet concentrate is required for 10 kg of body weight. For example, for an adult weighting 70 kg, 7 single donor units (containing at least × 10^9) per units are required which should raise the platelet count by 20–40 × 10^9/L. The increase in platelet count will be relatively less in cases of splenomegaly, septicemia, and disseminated intravascular coagulation (DIC) (Box 5.14).

All platelet components are leukodepleted and irradiated prior to release to the hospital.

5.6.2 Apheresis Platelets in Platelet Additive Solution (PAS)

Dose of platelets obtained from a single donor and suspended in a mixture of PAS and 40% donor plasma. Apheresis platelets indicated in cases that require repeated transfusion such as in cases of aplastic anemia in order to reduce the risk of alloimmunization (Box 5.15).

5.6.3 Pediatric Apheresis Platelets in PAS (Pedipaks)

One unit of apheresis platelets may be divided into three equal packs to create pediatric-sized components (pedipaks). This will enable smaller patients requiring small but regular top-ups to have exposure to less donor products and minimize product wastage (Box 5.16).

Box 5.14: Showing Types of Platelets

Apheresis platelets in platelet additive solution (PAS)
Pediatric apheresis platelets in PAS (pedipaks)
Pooled platelets in PAS

5.6.4 Pooled Platelets in PAS

An adult dose of pooled platelets is obtained from a pool of buffy coats from four donors. These are pooled and resuspended in PAS to create 1 unit of pooled platelets.

Patient with mild to moderate allergic reaction to apheresis platelets may require pooled platelets as the first choice. The ratio of plasma to platelets is less in pooled components than apheresis products, and therefore the exposure to plasma is less (Box 5.17).

5.6.5 Compatibility

ABO compatibility is desirable but not essential in case of platelet transfusion. In absence of group-specific compatibility of available platelets,

Box 5.15: Showing Characteristics of Apheresis Platelets

Volume (mL): 198 ± 11 (100–400 mL)
Platelet count (10^9/unit) 274 ± 31

Box 5.16: Showing Characteristics of Pediatric Apheresis Platelets in PAS (pedipaks)

Volume (mL): 54 ± 3 (40–60 mL)
Platelet count (10^9/unit) 68 ± 6

Box 5.17: Showing Characteristics of Pooled Platelets

Volume (mL) 326 ± 14 (>160)
Platelet count(10^9/unit) 284 ± 40

patient's clinical condition, urgency of treatment, age, sex, weight, and diagnosis should be considered for transfusion.

Infusion of group O platelets to group A patient may be associated with clinically significant transfusion reactions, including a positive DAT, red cell hemolysis, and even lower platelet survival.

Platelet components contain a small number of red cells and for this reason female with childbearing potential should be given only Rh-compatible platelet transfusion; if it is unavoidable, consider giving Rhesus immunoglobulin.

5.6.6 Platelet Swirling Phenomenon

The presence of the swirling phenomenon is useful to define platelet or platelet-rich plasma that is suitable for transfusion. The viable platelets in an "unactivated" state have a discoid appearance, and that shape causes light to be scattered in multiple different directions creating a cloud- or swirl-like appearance. Platelets that are activated in a low pH environment lose their discoid shape and lose their light-scattering abilities. Results of a platelet swirling test are recorded as positive or extensive swirl, moderate or intermediate swirl, and absent or negative swirl.

Platelet agitator with built-in incubator is essential equipment in maintaining a temperature of +22 ± 2 °C. Platelet incubator provides a compact digitally controlled and closely monitored environment for **platelet incubation and storage** conditions. This equipment is available in small units for laboratory use as well as large floor models for maximum capacity. These incubators include built-in agitators, motion failure alarms, and circular chart recorders to provide optimal condition for the storage of platelets. One of them is PF15i agitator with a capacity of up to 15 random bags, or 5 apheresis bags, set on perforated shelving that will rock sample bags side to side on smooth glide. Delrin acetal resin rollers provide high tensile strength, creep resistance, and toughness. When the door to this **benchtop shaking incubator** is opened, the agitator pauses and then automatically resumes once the door is closed.

Amplitude of the platelet agitator: The side-to-side movement of the tray of the platelet agitator is expected to be within the range of 3.6–4.0 cm.

Stroke: 65–75 strokes per minute (the number of times the tray of the platelet agitator moves from side to side per minute).

Storage of platelets: Length of time permitted for the storage and transportation of platelet concentrates within the temperature range +20 to +24 °C (Table 5.6).

Platelet concentrates are prepared from whole blood by differential centrifugation. In this process the red cells are first separated at low speed followed by high speed centrifugation for sedimenting platelets.

The survival time of platelets with in the body is 2–6 days, and daily transfusions are usually needed. When platelets are given to a bleeding patient, the therapeutic effect is measured by improved hemostasis, and not by the improvement in laboratory values of the platelet count.

5.7 Medicine and Transfusion Options

Chronic renal failure: Recombinant erythropoietin is preferred.

5.7.1 Recombinant Erythropoietin

In normal person the new red blood cells (RBCs) are generated at a rate of 2.5 million per second from the bone marrow to replenish the continuous removal of effete RBCs. The production of RBCs (erythropoiesis) is controlled by an intricate interaction between various humoral factors and cytokines. Erythropoietin is essential for

Table 5.6 Showing storage temperature of platelets

Process	Maximum storage time
Storage	5 days
Transport	24 h
After issue, before transfusion	30 min
Open system and/or pooled	4 h

proliferation, differentiation & maturation of RBC in bome marrow.

There is increasing evidence that RHuEPO can minimize the need for blood transfusion in patients requiring cardiothoracic or any major surgery.

In patients who were not eligible for autologous donation, a low dose of RHuEPO (150 IU/kg/week) given 3–4 weeks before surgery reduced the blood transfusion requirement by nearly 50%.

The treatment with RHuEPO is only applicable in non-acute or planned situation.

The most common side effect of RHuEPO is "flu-like" syndrome. It is usually mild in nature and subsides with simple supportive measures with in 24 h.

Disorder of hemostasis: Vitamin K is the treatment of choice for hemorrhagic disease of the new born, and transfusion is usually not indicated.

Identification and correction of the underlying cause is key stone in the management of patients with DIC.

Blood component specific to the disorder is preferred to whole blood.

Crystalloids, physiological saline, and Ringer's lactate can effectively correct hypovolemia even in massive injury. The crystalloids rapidly diffuse into the interstitial fluid space; therefore the volume administered should be about three times the estimated blood loss.

Side effects of crystalloid infusion

A fraction of the infused crystalloid passes into the interstitial space and may cause tissue edema. Transient tissue edema is acceptable except in patients with severe anemia or cardiopulmonary dysfunctions. Even large volumes of crystalloids used for resuscitation rarely produce pulmonary edema in the absence of heart failure.

Synthetic colloids: Colloid solutions exert an oncotic pressure because of macromolecules they contain; this retains water and thus volume in circulation.

Types of synthetic colloids are:

Dextran and HES (6%) are true plasma expanders. The volume expansion with dextran 70 and HES has more prolonged effect than that of gelatins.

The colloids (hydroxyethyl starch, dextran, or gelatin) are retained within the circulation for longer periods (4–8 h). They are potentially life-saving fluids.

Dextran 70 is used to treat cases of hypovolemia (decreased volume of circulating blood plasma) that can result from surgery, trauma or injury, severe burns, or other causes of bleeding.

Side effects:

- Allergic reactions: skin rash and hives
- Swelling on face, tongue, lips, or throat
- Swelling or bruising along the vein where the medicine was injected
- Chest tightness, weak or shallow breathing, or a light-headed feeling Nausea, vomiting, joint pain; fever; or pain

Dextran 40 is given prophylactically indicated to reduce the incidence of post operative thromboembolism. It is also used in the adjunctive treatment of shock or impending shock due to hemorrhage, burns, surgery, or other trauma. It is not indicated as a replacement for whole blood or blood components if they are available.

HES (Hespan) is (6% hetastarch in 0.9% sodium chloride) Injection, solution.

Indications: In the treatment of hypovolemia when plasma volume expansion is desired. It is not a substitute for blood or plasma.

Hespan is administered by intravenous infusion only. Total dosage and rate of infusion depend upon the amount of blood or plasma lost and the resultant hemoconcentration. In critically ill adult patients, including patients with sepsis, use of hydroxyethyl starch (HES) products, including Hespan, increases risk of mortality and renal replacement therapy.

Contraindication: Critically ill adult patients including patients with sepsis.

HES interfere with hemostatic mechanism through the less than dextran.

Succinylated gelatin Gelofusine (B. Braun) is **4% solution in 500 and 1000 mL containers.**

An infusion of succinylated gelatin retains fluid in the intravascular space. The effect lasts for 3–4 h.

Indications: Plasma volume substitute.

In the treatment of hypovolemia due to bleeding.

The infusion can also be used when hemodilution or extracorporeal circulation is needed.

Albumin: Albumin (human) 5% and 25% is a sterile aqueous solution for intravenous use containing the albumin component human plasma. The solution is approximately isotonic and isooncotic with human plasma. The effective oncotic pressure of the solution depends largely on its albumin content.

Choice of 5% vs 25% depends on whether patient requires primarily volume (5%) or primarily protein/oncotic pressure (25%).

Indications: Albumin (human) 5% may be useful in the early therapy of shock associated with acute hemorrhagic pancreatitis and peritonitis. It has been found that the correction of the blood volume deficit and adequate fluid therapy is mandatory in the acute stage of pancreatitis and peritonitis when there is loss of fluid into the peritoneal cavity or the retroperitoneal space.

Hypoalbuminemia secondary to paracentesis for ascites.

Other indications are:

Post burn of severe degree after 24 h for chronic fluid replacement.

Immediate therapy during the first 24 h is directed at the administration of large volumes of crystalloid solutions and lesser amounts of albumin (human) 25% solution to maintain an adequate plasma volume and protein (colloid) content. For continuation of therapy beyond 24 h, larger amounts of albumin 25% and lesser amounts of crystalloid are generally used.

Used in patients with hypotension who has already received several liters of crystalloids and has not responded.

Used in conjunction with a diuretic in hypoproteinemic patient to remove excess IV fluids.

Preferable to FFP as volume expander in cases of burns.

Conditions for which albumin (human) 5% is usually not recommended:

Post operative albumin loss
Hypoproteinemia with an oncotic deficit

Contraindication: History of adverse reaction with previous albumin transfusion.

In patients with pulmonary edema, cardiac failure, or severe anemia because of the risk of acute circulatory overload.

Upon administration of albumin (human) 5%, there is a rapid increase of the plasma volume about equal to the volume infused. The initial dose for adults is 250–500 mL. The quantity given may be increased to a total of 0.5 g albumin per pound of body weight (i.e., 10 mL/pound), but administration should be monitored by careful observation.

It is available in 5% and 25% solution. It can be given without regard to ABO and Rh grouping and without crossmatch. Its primary function is volume expander. Albumin expands the vascular space for a longer period than electrolyte solution.

Saline and Ringer lactate expand the entire extravascular fluid space.

Colloids expand intravascular volume more than crystalloids. It means smaller amount of colloid is required for adequate intravascular resuscitation.

It can be stored for 5 years at 2–10 °C. It is free from transmission of HIV and hepatitis B virus.

Further Reading

BS/EN/ISO 1135-4. Transfusion equipment for medical use—part 4: transfusion sets for single use.

EN/ISO 15223-1:2007/Amendment A1:2008. Medical devices—symbols to be used with medical device labels, labelling and information to be supplied—part general requirements. Archived from https://www.iso.org/standard/45420.html.

Hod EA, Francis RO, Spitalnik SL. RBC storage lesion-induced adverse effects: more smoke; is there fire? Anesth Analg. 2017;124(6):1752.

Sharma S, Sharma P, Tyler LN. Transfusion of blood and blood products: indications and complications. Am Fam Physician. 2011;83(6):719–24.

Sparrow RL. Red blood cell storage and transfusion-related immunomodulation. Blood Transfus. 2010;8(Suppl 3):s26.

Standards Australia on behalf of Committee HE-020. AS 3864.2-2012 Medical refrigeration equipment—for the storage of blood and blood products—user related requirements for care, maintenance, performance verification and calibration, NSW, 2012. Archived from https://www.blood.gov.au/australian-standards-38642-2012.

Standards Australia on behalf of Committee HE-020. AS 3864.1-2012 Medical refrigeration equipment—for the storage of blood and blood products—manufacturing requirements, NSW, 2012. Archived from https://infostore.saiglobal.com/en-us/standards/as-3864-1-2012-120205_saig_as_as_251937/#:~:text=Specifies%20requirements%20for%20the%20manufacture,25%C2%B0C%20or%20lower.

Zimring JC. Fresh versus old blood: are there differences and do they matter? Hematology. 2013;2013(1):651–5.

6 Blood Component Preparation

6.1 General Principles of Component Preparation

Blood is a life-saving liquid organ. It is a mixture of cells, colloids, and crystalloids that can be separated into different blood components, namely, packed red blood cell (pRBC) or red cell concentrate (RCC), platelet concentrate, fresh frozen plasma, and cryoprecipitate. As different blood components have different relative density, sediment rate, and size, they can be separated when centrifugal force is applied. Each blood component is used for a specific indication; thus the component separation has maximized the utility of one whole blood unit. Different components need different storage conditions and temperature requirements for therapeutic efficacy.

The donor blood is collected as 350 or 450 mL in double, triple, quadruple, or penta bags with CPDA-1 or additive solution. After blood collection, components should be separated within 5–8 h. Component room should be a separate sanitized room. All precautions to avoid red cell contamination have to be taken such as tapping the segment ends, proper balancing of opposite bags, and following standard programs and protocols described in the manual of refrigerated centrifuge manufacturer. The program is run with mainly two spins—heavy spin (e.g., 5000 G for 10–15 min) and light spin (e.g., 1500 G for 5–7 min). The heavy and light spin configuration vary with manufacturer and model. Here "G" is relative centrifugal force calculated using revolutions per minute and rotor length. Use of totally automated component separator instrument will allow for the preparation of low-volume blood components with a recovery of 90% of whole blood platelets.

6.2 Laboratory Procedures in Blood Component Preparation

The whole blood (350–450 mL) is collected from a healthy donor, in primary bag (No. 1) having satellites bag double, triple, quadruple or penta bags with CPDA-1 or additive solution.

Venipuncture should be clean with minimum trauma.

Flow of blood should be rapid and uninterrupted.

During collection, agitate the bag in order to mix the blood adequately with anticoagulant.

After blood collection, components should be separated within 5–8 h.

P. S. Ajmani, *Immunohematology and Blood banking*, https://doi.org/10.1007/978-981-15-8435-0_6

6.3 Preparation of Fresh Frozen Plasma and Packed Red Cells

Collect blood in a double blood bag with ACD, and store in the refrigerator at 4 °C until processed which would be within 4 h.

Put the bags into plastic overlaps and place in the centrifuge cups. Balance the bags accurately with the same amount of other bag.

Load the centrifuge and spin at 5000 G for 10 min at 5 °C.

Remove about 2/3 volume of plasma into satellite bag.

Seal the tubing and separate the bags.

Label the plasma bag as **fresh frozen plasma.**

Indicate the date of preparation on the bag.

Place the plasma in cardboard cartoon and store in the freezer at −30 °C or lower. Other method is to put a rubber band around the bag before freezing to crimp the bag. When the bag thaws, crimping disappears. The primary bag containing the red cell is labeled as **packed red blood cell** (Table 6.1).

6.4 Additive Solutions

All of the currently licensed RBC additive solutions have an acidic pH (5.6–5.8), which is well below the normal physiological pH of 7.3 of venous blood. Acidic additive solutions (and anticoagulants) are used simply because it is easier to heat-sterilize a glucose-containing solution at an acidic pH. Nevertheless, during storage RBCs undergo a complex and progressive accumulation of physiochemical changes, collectively referred to as the RBC storage lesion (Box 6.1).

6.5 Preparation of Cryoprecipitate

To prepare cryoprecipitate, a three-bag arrangement (one primary bag and two satellite bags) is required.

Collect the FFP in the first satellite bag. The second satellite bag will be used for the collection of cryoprecipitate. The primary bag contains the red cell concentrates that are kept separately.

Box 6.1: Showing Names of Additive Solutions

AS-1 Adosol
AS-3 Nutricell
AS-5
MAP
PAGGSM

Table 6.1 Showing shelf life of blood components

Component	Temp	Preservative	Shelf life
pRBCs	4 °C	CPDA	35 days
pRBCs, apheresis		Additive solution	42 days
pRBCs leucodepleted		Additive solution	42 days
Apheresis + leucodepleted	4 °C	Open	24 h
RBC irradiated	4 °C		28 days
RBC irradiated[a]	4 °C		24 h
Saline washed	4 °C		24 h
Frozen RBCs	−65 °C	40% glycerol	10 years
Frozen RBCs	−120 °C	20% glycerol	10 years
Deglycerolized RBCS	4 °C	Open system	24 h
		Closed system	14 days
Rejuvenated RBCs	4 °C	CPDA-1	24 h
	4 °C	Additive solution	42 days
Washed rejuvenated	4 °C		24 h
Deglycerolized rejuvenated	4 °C		24 h
Frozen rejuvenated	−65 °C		10 years

[a]In neonates in order to avoid hyperkalemia, the shelf life of irradiated RBC is 24 h only

Proceed with the FFP for cryoprecipitate preparation.

Place the frozen bag (No. 2) of plasma and attach empty satellite bag (No. 3) in a 2–4 °C cold room for about 1 h.

When the blood bag is no longer brittle, hang the bag with the frozen plasma (No. 2) in an inverted position with ports lowermost. Place the satellite bag (No. 3) on a lower shelf.

Allow the thawed plasma to flow from the primary plasma bag (No. 2) to the satellite bag (No. 3). Observe periodically to make sure that the thawing plasma is not accumulating in the primary bag (No. 2). The cryoprecipitate remains enmeshed in the frozen plasma in the primary bag (No. 2); when the primary plasma bag (No. 2) weighs approximately 30 g, the tubing between the bags is sealed, and the two bags are separated. The bag (No. 2) of cryoprecipitate is labeled and stored at −30 °C or lower.

The satellite bag (No. 3) containing the thawed plasma is labeled as **single-unit plasma** and stored in the refrigerator at 2–4 °C.

6.6 Reconstitution of Cryoprecipitate for Transfusion

The cryoprecipitate is reconstituted by the blood bank technician and then issued for transfusion.

The procedure is as follows:

Thaw the required number of bags with cryoprecipitate by placing them in an overwrap in a 37 °C water bath. After thawing a gelatinous white residue will remain. It is called cryoprecipitate as it forms in cold conditions.

The entry port should remain above the water level.

The cryoprecipitate should dissolve in 30 min. Gentle kneading may be necessary to completely dissolve it. Should some cryoprecipitate remain undissolved, addition of a small volume of sterile saline will dissolve it. Pool the thawed cryoprecipitate from all the bags into one bag, and wash out each bag with 10 mL of saline which is added to the pooled cryoprecipitate. Label bag and indicate the number of units of cryoprecipitate pooled in it.

Cryoprecipitate is a labile plasma component that cannot be kept at room temperature for more than 4 h.

Cryoprecipitate is a concentrate of high molecular weight plasma proteins. From 1 unit of whole blood (450), 80 to 100 IU of factor VIII are obtained in a volume of 10–15 mL which also contains approximately 250 mg of fibrinogen. The concentrate contains factor VIII (antihemophilic factor), von Willebrand factor (vWF), fibrinogen, factor XIII, fibronectin, and small amounts of other plasma proteins.

The commercial preparation of cryoprecipitate is in lyophilized form. The non-lyophilized cryoprecipitate must be stored below 30 °C for optimal stability, while the lyophilized vials can be stored at 4 °C.

Cryodepleted plasma ("cryosupernatant") is the plasma supernatant that remains following removal of the cryoprecipitate from frozen–thawed plasma. It contains all the other plasma proteins and clotting factors present in plasma that remain soluble during cold-temperature thawing of the plasma.

6.7 Preparation of Platelet-Rich Plasma (PRP)

Collect blood in ACD in triple bag and keep at 20 °C until processed. Do not refrigerate.

Load the centrifuge as described under FFP preparation, and leave the bag (No. 1) primary undisturbed for 60 min at 20–22 °C.

Then centrifuge the bags at 1500 G for 10 min.

Remove 2/3 volume of plasma into satellite bag (No. 2).

Seal the tubing between the bags and separate the two bags. If platelet concentrate is to be made, do not seal the tubes or separate the bags; instead, apply a temporary seal by means of a rubber band on the tubing until the platelet concentrate is made.

Label the satellite bag (No. 2) as **platelet-rich plasma** which is stored at 20–22 °C until issued for transfusion. The primary bag is labeled as **packed red cells.**

6.8 Preparation of Platelet Concentrates

Centrifuge the platelet-rich plasma (PR) of the satellite bag (No. 2) at 2500 G for 20 min. The upper layer of the plasma (supernatant) contains platelet-poor plasma, and the lower layer is the plasma with most of the platelets.

Remove the platelet-poor plasma into second satellite bag (No. 3) or into original bag leaving approximately 50 mL of plasma with the platelet.

Seal the tubing and separate the bag with platelet concentrate (No. 2).

Leave the bag of platelet concentrate undisturbed for 60 min at 20–22 °C.

At the end of the period, suspend the platelets by gentle agitation of the bag for about 15 min.

Label the bag as platelet concentrate and store at 20–22 °C (room temperature) under gentle agitation. Platelets have a shelf life of 72 h if stored at room temperature with constant slow agitation; this is because the platelets have the tendency to aggregate.

The platelet-poor plasma is labeled as **single-unit plasma** and stored in the refrigerator.

6.9 Preparation of pRBC

This component is obtained by removing most of the plasma after centrifuging whole blood collected into anticoagulant.

Red cells may be resuspended in other additives to prolong storage and are filtered to remove most leucocytes.

A red cell unit is divided into four packs of equal volume to create Red cells Paediatric Leucocyte Depleted Units to minimize product wastage.

Washed leucocyte-depleted red cells are prepared by using a manual process by washing with saline–adenine–glucose–mannitol (SAGM) solution to remove the majority of plasma proteins, antibodies, and electrolytes.

Further Reading

Branch DR, Judd WJ, Johnson ST, Storry JR. Judd's methods in immunohematology. Bethesda, MD: AABB Press; 2008.

Burnouf T, Su CY, Radosevich M, Goubran H, El-Ekiaby M. Blood-derived biomaterials: fibrin sealant, platelet gel and platelet fibrin glue. ISBT Sci Ser. 2009;4(1):136–42.

Faber JC. Blood cold chain. ISBT Sci Ser. 2007;2(2):1–6.

Hardwick J. Blood processing. ISBT Sci Ser. 2008;3(2):148–76.

Hardwick J. Blood storage and transportation. ISBT Sci Ser. 2008;3(2):177–96.

Hillyer C, Hillyer KL, Strobl F, Jefferies L, Silberstein L, editors. Handbook of transfusion medicine. San Diego, CA: Academic Press; 2001.

James V, McClelland B. Guidelines for the blood transfusion services in the United Kingdom. London: The Stationery Office; 2005.

Klein HG. Immunology of red cells. In: Klein HG, Anstee DJ, editors. Mollison's blood transfusion in clinical medicine. Oxford: Wiley Blackwell; 2014.

Letowska M. Patient-specific component requirements: 'right blood, right patient, right time, right place'. ISBT Sci Ser. 2009;4(1):52–5.

Lotens A, Najdovski T, Cellier N, Ernotte B, Lambermont M, Rapaille A. New approach to 'top-and-bottom' whole blood separation using the multiunit TACSI WB system: quality of blood components. Vox Sang. 2014;107(3):261–8.

Moog R. A new technology in blood collection: multicomponent apheresis. In: New developments in blood transfusion research. New York: Nova Science Publishers, Inc.; 2006. p. 141–6.

Simon TL, McCullough J, Snyder EL, Solheim BG, Strauss RG, editors. Rossi's principles of transfusion medicine. Chichester: John Wiley & Sons; 2016.

Sweeney JD, Rizk Y. Clinical transfusion medicine. Austin, TX: Landes Bioscience; 1999.

Wares F, Balasubramanian R, Mohan A, Sharma SK. Extrapulmonary tuberculosis: management and control. New Delhi: Directorate General of Health Services, Ministry of Health & Family Welfare; 2005. p. 95–114.

7 Blood Test in Immunohematology and Blood Banking

7.1 Collection of Blood Specimen

Collect 3 mL of blood in screw-capped plain test tube of 12 × 75 mm without any anticoagulant for adults and 2 mL in EDTA tube.

For infants and children, collect between 250 mU and 1 mL of blood in vacutainer in mL of blood in vacutainer in (EDTA) tube (BD Microtainer). Invert the tube 8–10 times for proper mixing of blood with anticoagulant. The amount of blood to be taken from infant depends on his body weight. Extreme care should be taken while processing infant's blood sample for immunohematology and blood banking procedures. Any left sample should be preserved at 4 °C for other investigation.

Alternatively infant's sample can also be taken in plain tube (without any anticoagulant) (white top) in order to avoid hemolysis.

Keep the infant blood sample at room temperature till the clot forms and then centrifuged at low speed of 500 rpm till the serum sample is clearly obtained.

Removal of more than 10% of an infant's blood volume in a short period of time can lead to serious consequences, such as iatrogenic anemia or cardiac arrest.

For adults, allow (tube for adult) it to stand for 30 min or till clot forms.

Centrifuge the clotted specimen (adult) at 1500 rpm for 5 min, and separate the serum into another previously labeled test tube.

Cells are separated from the clot with the help of Pasteur pipette, and suspend red cells in saline in another prelabeled test tube.

Use red cell suspension in forward grouping and serum for reverse grouping.

Hemolyzed samples are not suitable for testing.

The samples should be stored at 4 °C and preferably be tested within 48 h.

7.2 Blood Sample Handling and Processing

Pre-centrifugation handling: The first critical step in the laboratory testing process, after obtaining the sample, is the preparation of the blood samples. Specimen integrity can be maintained by following some basic handling processes:

Fill tubes to the stated draw volume to ensure the proper blood-to-additive ratio.

Allow the tubes to fill up to the specification of the tube.

Vacutainer tubes should be stored at 4–25 °C (39–77 °F).

Tubes should not be used beyond the designated expiration date.

P. S. Ajmani, *Immunohematology and Blood banking*, https://doi.org/10.1007/978-981-15-8435-0_7

Mix all gel barrier and additive tubes by gentle inversion five to ten times immediately after the draw. This assists in the clotting process. This also assures homogenous mixing of the additives with the blood in all types of additive tubes.

Keep the unclotted tubes in a vertical position for 30 min at room temperature. If the tubes are centrifuged early, the sample will get hemolyzed. Short clotting times can result in fibrin formation, which may interfere with complete gel barrier formation.

Preparation of reagent cells for blood grouping: The ratio of serum to red cells may affect the sensitivity of agglutination tests, and 5% red cell suspension is most suitable in most of the immunological procedures.

Reagent cells are needed to identify corresponding antibodies. Three types of reagent cells are needed to identify the corresponding antibodies related to ABO group—A cells, B cells, and O cells. Blood group AB can also be included, but not essential. Identify three different donors with known blood group of A, B, and O each.

- **Group A cells**: Collect 2 mL blood of three different group A donors in plain tube without any anticoagulant, and label them as A1, A2, and A3 tubes including A_1 subtype. Cells are obtained from the bottom of the clotted blood. EDTA anticoagulated sample may be the second choice.
- **Group B cells**: Similarly collect 2 mL blood of three different B group donors, and label them as B1, B2, and B3 tubes.
- **Group O cells**: Also collect 2 mL blood of three different group O donors, and label them as O1, O2, and O3 tubes.

Label three 12 × 75 mm tubes as A, B, and O.

Transfer 5 drops of red cells each from all the 3 different A group sample tubes into the A tube (total 15 drops, approximately 1 mL).

Similarly transfer 5 drops of red cells each from all the B group blood sample into the B tube (total 15 drops, approximately 1 mL).

Transfer 5 drops of red cells each from all the three different group O sample tubes into the O tube (total 15 drops, approximately 1 mL).

Fill all the three tubes with ¾ of normal saline to suspend the cells and centrifuge at 1500 rpm for 5 min.

Wash the cells three times with normal saline.

Resuspend the cell button thoroughly between each wash, before adding more saline to ensure complete washing.

The last wash should always have a clear supernatant with no signs of hemolysis.

After the last washing, decant the supernatant leaving packed red cell suspension in the bottom of the tube.

Prepare 5% red cell suspension in saline for the tube method and 10% for the slide method.

7.2.1 Preparation of Reagent O Cells for Antibody Screening

Reagent O red cells are used for the detection of irregular or abnormal antibodies other than the once associated with ABO group.

7.2.1.1 Procedure

Identify and select four different group O Rh-positive donors. Collect 2 mL blood from each donor in plain test tube without any anticoagulant. Allow the blood to clot at 37 °C for 30 min.

Remove the cells from the clot, and suspend the specimens individually in saline, and wash the cells four times as mentioned in the above procedure.

Pool the washed cells of two donors together in equal ratio of five drops each.

Repeat the same for the other two donors.

Label these two groups of pooled O-positive cells as I and II.

These pooled O-positive cells will be used for the antibody screening but not for identification. Identification of specific antibody can only be done by using O cells with known antigenic characters also known as panel cells. These antigenic characters are established by reference laboratories after reacting them with known antibodies.

7.2.2 Preparation of Coombs Control Cells or Sensitized Cells

Coombs control cells are **"sensitized" O-positive cells**. Sensitization of O-positive cells is brought about by reacting them with weak anti-D in a way that the O-positive cells are coated with anti-D (IgG), but the immunologic reaction is not strong enough to bring agglutination. These sensitized O-positive cells agglutinate when they come in contact with antihuman globulin or Coombs serum.

Usage of Coombs control cells: These are used to test the reactivity of antihuman globulin serum or Coombs reagent. This is crucial in the final stage of crossmatching (AHG) phase. Lack of hemagglutination in the AHG phase of crossmatching could indicate compatible red cells of donor with the antibodies of the recipient present in the serum. This negative hemagglutination can also be a false indication of compatibility due to the use of inactive AHG. In order to eliminate the latter, add sensitized O-positive cells into the tube with AHG and 5% suspension of donor's red cells; the sensitized cells must agglutinate, indicating that the AHG is active.

7.2.3 Preparation of Coombs Control Cells

Bring all the reagents to room temperature (25–30 °C) before testing.

7.2.3.1 Procedure

Take a glass tube 12 × 75 mm, and collect 2 mL of O Rh (D)-positive blood in EDTA tube, and mix it well by inversion.

Transfer 1 mL of the sample in another tube, and add 5 mL of normal saline, and centrifuge at 1500 rpm for 10 min.

Decant the supernatant after the first wash and repeat washing three times with normal saline.

The last wash should always have a clear supernatant with no signs of hemolysis. If it shows sign of hemolysis, repeat the procedure with 1 mL of left blood.

After the last washing, decant the supernatant and suspend the red cells in 0.5 mL of normal saline. Now add three drops of anti-D and mix. Observe the reaction macroscopically. The 1+ reaction is recognized by the formation of a few clumps with many free cells and a turbid background. If the anti-D brings more than 1+ agglutination reaction, anti-D should be further diluted.

Incubate the Rh-positive cells suspended in weak anti-D at 37 °C for 15 min. The cells get sensitized with anti-D coating.

After incubation wash the sensitized red blood cells thoroughly five times with 5 mL of normal saline with repeated centrifugation.

After the last washing, decant the supernatant, and prepare a 5% suspension of the sensitized red cells by adding saline to the packed cell in ratio of 2.5 and 0.1 mL.

Take a drop of sensitized cell suspension in a test tube and add antihuman globin reagent; mix and centrifuge for 1 min at 1000 rpm or 20 s at 3400 rpm. Very gently resuspend the cell button and observe for agglutination macroscopically the agglutination reaction. It should give 4+ reaction.

Interpretation: Agglutination indicates that the red cells are sensitized and the antihuman globulin serum is functional and the test is valid.

A negative reaction of AHG is confirmed by adding sensitized O cells. Agglutination indicates the presence of active AHG, and the negative reaction in the previous step is truly negative, and not due to the inactivation of AHG reagent.

A stabilized suspension of 5% Coombs control cells is thus prepared, and store the Coombs

Table 7.1 Showing interpretation of macroscopic agglutination reaction in the test tube

Observation	Report
One solid aggregate, clear background	4+
2–3 large agglutinates with clear background	3+
Several small agglutinates, many free cells, clear background	2+
Several small agglutinates, reddish background of free cells	1+
Tiny aggregates, turbid background giving a granular appearance	W
No agglutination or hemolysis (negative)	O
Mixture of agglutinated + unagglutinated red cells	Mf
Complete hemolysis (positive)	H
Partial hemolysis + some unhemolyzed red cells	PH

control cells at 2–8 °C. Use within 4 weeks of preparation (Table 7.1).

Hemolysis (pink color of the supernatant after centrifugation) should be considered as positive immunologic reaction between the red cell antigen and the corresponding antibody.

7.2.4 Reporting of Hemagglutination Reaction

Antibody can be detected in the serum of humans; if the red cells are used as a source of antigen, the assay is called hemagglutination.

Antibody is measured by hemagglutination at lower concentrations than those detectable by other techniques. This relies on the ability of antibody to cross-link red blood cells by interacting with the antigens on their surface.

The agglutination of an antigen, as a result of cross-linking by antibodies, is dependent on the correct proportion of antigen to antibody. Hemagglutination is expressed as titer: it is the inverse of the last dilution that is positive; e.g., 1/1000. It helps to assess the degree of immunologic reaction and is also useful in the determination of titer.

ABO blood group and Rh group are the first steps of laboratory procedure before proceeding for the crossmatching of recipient's blood with group compatible donor's blood. ABO systems are necessary to identify suitable blood components for transfusion.

Blood group refers to the entire blood group system comprising red blood cell (RBC) antigens whose specificity is controlled by a series of genes which can be allelic or linked very closely on the same chromosome.

Blood type refers to a specific pattern of reaction to testing antisera within a given system over a period of time.

7.3 Blood Group Typing

In routine clinical analysis, there is a wide range of established procedures and practices for blood typing, where nearly all of them deal with the formation of agglutinates. There is a wide range of blood typing techniques which differ from each other in terms of sensitivity, reagents and equipment required, the time of operation, and analysis. Two basic methods to observe the hemagglutination reaction in ABO blood grouping and Rh typing are the slide and test tube method with their inbuilt advantages and drawbacks.

The slide test has good sensitive method among others, for blood group determination, and due to its prompt results, it widely acceptable and valuable in emergency and routine cases.

In comparison to the slide test, the tube test is more sensitive and reliable; therefore, it can be used conveniently for blood transfusion crossmatching procedure and when sufficient time is available for testing. In this method, both forward (cell) and reverse (serum) grouping are carried out.

Among other methods, microplate technology is a further step toward more sensitive and fast blood typing analysis with the feasibility of automation. In this technique, both antibodies in blood plasma and antigens on RBCs can be determined.

Methods of determination of ABO blood grouping: ABO grouping is done in two ways—forward grouping and reverse grouping.

Forward grouping suggests the presence or absence of A and B antigens in RBCs.

Reverse grouping indicates the presence or absences of anti-A and anti-B antibodies in serum.

Principle of forward grouping: A suspension of red cells of the test specimen is reacted with known anti-A and anti-B sera. Positive agglutination indicates the presence of corresponding antigen (agglutinogen) on the red cells.

Principle of reverse grouping: Serum of the test sample is reacted with known A and B cells. Agglutination indicates the presence of corresponding antibody in serum.

The forward and reverse reaction should be compatible with each other in determination of the blood group. In absence of I,t, look for the possible technical error or the presence of subgroups.

7.3.1 Preparation of Red Cell Suspension

Principle: A red cell suspension is needed for all hemagglutination tests. Red cell suspensions provide the appropriate serum to cell ratio to allow for grading and interpretation of test results.

7.3.1.1 Why Red Cell Wash Is Necessary

A proper ratio of plasma to red cells is important for accuracy in antigen–antibody reactions; too heavy a concentration of cells might result in a weak or false negative reaction.

Abnormal patient albumin: Globulin ratios may cause pseudoagglutination, so adequate washing is important in the preparation of the cell suspension.

Before washing, soluble antigens such as A and B may be present, which can interfere in test results?

Wharton's jelly, which is present in newborn's cord blood, may affect the agglutination reaction.

Cold-acting autoimmune antibodies and increased levels of immunoglobulins may cause either agglutination or rouleaux.

Hemolyzed red blood cells due to a difficult draw will interfere in grading and interpretation of hemolysis.

Fibrinogen can result in fibrin strands forming that makes grading reactions difficult.

The cells must be washed 4–5 times with large volume (5 mL) of normal saline, in order to remove plasma. Weak cell suspensions are used in hemagglutination tests, since the ratio of serum to cells affects the sensitivity of most tests—a minimum number of antibodies must bound to RBCs in order to bring about agglutination.

Clotted blood or anticoagulated blood must be washed in normal saline to remove the contaminated antibodies. Finally the requisite strength of red cell suspensions is made in saline.

7.3.1.2 Procedure for Cell Washing

Take a 12 × 75 mm glass tube and label the tubes as per serial number of samples or patient's name.

Add 1 mL whole blood (anticoagulated) or 1 mL of coagulated blood (from the bottom of the test tube) and 8 mL of normal saline by positioning the tip of the wash bottle directly over the tube and squeezing it. This will mix the blood and the saline, increasing the efficiency of washing. Avoid contamination of tubes when dispensing saline into several tubes.

Since antibody-coated RBCs are heavier than uncoated cells and settle to the bottom of the sample, the contents should be mixed well before blood is removed. If a clotted specimen is used, blood should be removed from the bottom of the clot for the same reason.

Centrifuge at 2500 rpm for 3 min at room temperature.

When the centrifuge stops, remove the test tube and decant the supernatant saline and discard.

Wash three times as above till supernatant saline is clear.

The last wash should always have a clear supernatant with no signs of hemolysis.

Consider red cell pellet as 100%. Shake the cells loose from the bottom of the tube.

Prepare red cell suspension as shown below (Tables 7.2 and 7.3):

Table 7.2 Showing red cell percentage by micropipette method

RBC %	1%	2%	3%	5%	10%	20%	45%
Saline	10 mL	10 mL	10 mL	10 mL	10 mL	10 mL	10 mL
PRBC	100 μL	200 μL	300 μL	500 μL	1000 μL	2000 μL	4500 μL

Table 7.3 Showing red cell percentage by drop method

RBC %	3%	5%	10%	20%	50%
Saline	32 drops	20 drops	10 drops	5 drops	5 drops
pRBC	1 drop	1 drop	1 drop	1 drop	5 drop

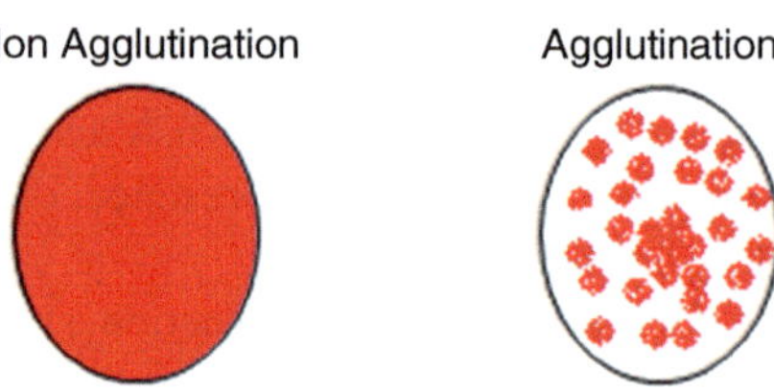

Fig. 7.1 Showing agglutination

7.3.2 ABO Grouping

Testing with both anti-A and anti-B is necessary to determine if red blood cells possess or lack A and/or B blood group antigens. Absence of agglutination is a negative test result, which indicates the corresponding antigen is not present and demonstrable. Agglutination of red blood cells with a given reagent is a positive test result, which indicates the presence of the corresponding antigen on the red blood cells (forward type). Blood transfusion requires a mandatory crossmatch test to examine the compatibility between donor and recipient blood groups. Generally, in all crossmatch tests, hemagglutination reaction of antibodies with erythrocyte antigens is carried out to monitor agglutination.

In routine clinical analysis, there is a wide range of established procedures and practices for blood typing, where nearly all of them deal with the formation of agglutinates (Fig. 7.1 and Box 7.1).

Box 7.1: Showing Blood Grouping Methods

Slide method
Tube method
Microwell plate
Gel or column technique
Solid Phase Red Cell Adherence Assay (SPRCA)

7.3.3 ABO and Rh Grouping Sera

The potency of any antisera deteriorates rapidly if kept for too long at ambient temperature; grouping sera should, therefore, be kept at 4 °C or as directed by the manufacturer when not in use. Frozen antisera must be completely thawed before use, and no refreezing should be done.

7.3.4 Different Types of Serum

- **Anti-A serum**: is obtained from B group individuals, since there is natural occurrence of anti-A agglutinins in their serum.
- **Anti-B serum**: is obtained from group A individuals where there is natural occurrence of anti-B antibody in the serum.
- **Anti-AB (monoclonal IgM)**: This is intended to use as a reagent for the detection of the "AB" antigen present on human red blood cell.
- **Anti-AB typing serum**: is obtained from group O individuals.

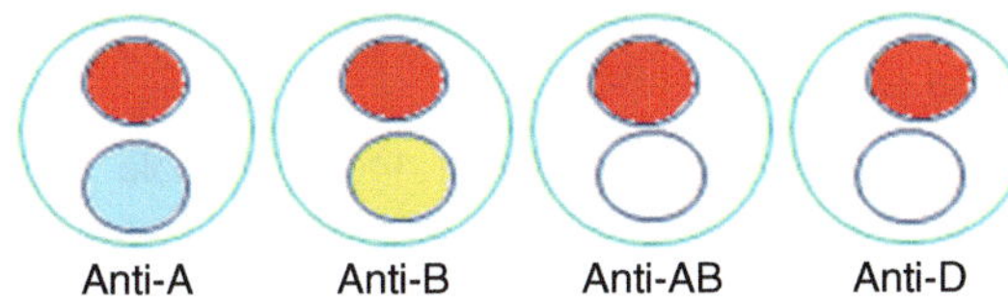

- **Anti-AB** human red blood cells possessing AB antigen will agglutinate when mixed with anti-AB antibody, directed toward AB antigen. Agglutination of red blood cells with anti-AB is a positive test reaction and indicates the presence of AB antigens on the RBCs. Absence of agglutination of red blood cells with anti-AB is a negative test result, and it indicates the absence of AB antigen on the RBCs.
- Anti-AB IgM.
- **Anti-A_1**: This serum is obtained from human sources or plant lectins.
- **Anti-H**: This serum is obtained from lectins, and antiserum is used for detection of Bombay (Oh) group.

Blend of IgM monoclonal + IgG polyclonal reagent: These antibodies are highly specific, react equally well at 20 °C as well as 37 °C, and are reliable for slide and rapid test tube technique.

IgM anti-D monoclonal reagent cannot be used for Du testing by indirect antiglobulin test (IAT), while IgM + IgG monoclonal reagent and blend of IgM monoclonal and IgG polyclonal can be used for Du testing.

ABO monoclonal and anti-D IgM reagents will give excellent results when diluted in phosphate buffer saline containing 1–3% bovine serum albumin.

Red cell suspension used for ABO and Rh grouping

Method	Red cell percentage (%)
ABO slide method	50
ABO tube method	5
ABO microplate method	1
ABO column or gel method	1
Rh slide method	50
Rh tube method	5

7.3.5 ABO Grouping Procedure by Slide Method

Take a clean glass slide and label two half of the same as A and B.

Add one drop of anti-A on the slide marked A and one drop of anti-B on the slide marked B. Hold the reagent dropper 1 inch above the slide to ensure a full drop is dispensed. **Do not** touch the dropper to the slide.

Add two drops of the 10% red cell suspension to both sections of the slide.

Mix the antiserum and cells with the help of toothpick or the corner of the other slide. Spread to form a 2 cm circle. Make sure the entire surface of the bottom of the circle is covered with the mixture.

Tilt the slide slowly, back and forth, for 2 min to complete the mixing.

Examine for agglutination within 2 min. Protect the slide for evaporation and drying particularly in hot weather. It may give erroneous results (Table 7.4).

Observation

Little clumps of red cells seen floating in clear liquid	Positive
No agglutination of red cells; cells are floating homogenously	Negative

Table 7.4 Report of forward grouping and probable blood group

Report of reaction with		
Anti-A	Anti-B	Probable blood groups
Positive	Negative	A
Negative	Positive	B
Positive	Positive	AB
Negative	Negative	O

No hemagglutination (negative) and hemagglutination (positive)

7.3.5.1 Disadvantages

- The slide method is less sensitive than the tube test.
- Drying up of the reaction mixture can cause aggregation of cells, giving false positive results.
- Weaker reactions are difficult to interpret.

7.3.6 Reverse or Serum Grouping by Slide Method

Serum reverse group may be unreliable in infants under 6 months. Antibodies detectable in the serum of infants prior to this age are most commonly of IgG type of maternal origin.

Take a microscopic slide and make three circles with glass marking pencil, or take a microscopic slide with three ceramic rings.

Label three circles as A, B, and O.

Prepare 10% red cell suspension of known A, B, and group O and label them separately.

Add one drop of known A red cell suspension in circle A.

Add one drop of known B red cell suspension in circle B.

Add one drop of known O red cell suspension in circle O.

Add two drops of test serum on the cell suspension on each circle.

Mix the serum with cell suspension with the help of toothpick or the corner of the slide. Spread over a 2 cm circle.

Observation: The agglutinates are usually smaller than those observed in forward grouping.

Considerable variations exist between individuals regarding the degree of reaction, which largely depends on the amount of anti-A and anti-B antibodies in the serum (Table 7.5).

7.3.6.1 Pitfalls in Reverse Grouping by Slide Method

Anti-A and anti-B antibodies are as weak as to be virtually undetected.

Certain atypical antibodies may be present and capable of reacting with antigens other than A or B, hence confusing the blood grouping.

Some A_2 or weaker subgroups of A have anti-A_1 along with anti-B in the serum and thus may react with both A and B cells (similar to group O).

Table 7.5 Report of reverse grouping and probable blood group

Agglutination reaction		Serum group	Probable group
A cells	B cells		
Negative	Positive	Anti-B	A
Positive	Negative	Anti-A	B
Negative	Negative	None	AB
Positive	Positive	Anti-A, Anti-B	O

7.3.7 Tube Test for Forward Grouping

ABO grouping should be done only at room temperature. The test is performed with either (1) washed 5% red cell suspension or by (2) whole anticoagulated blood.

The test procedure is the same in both the tests except that in whole blood a tiny drop of blood should be taken equivalent to 5% red cell suspension.

Arrange three test tubes (10 × 75 mm) and label them as A, B, and AB.

Add one drop of anti-A serum in the test tube marked "A."

Add one drop of anti-B serum in the tube marked as "B."

Add one drop of anti-AB serum in the tube marked as "AB."

Add two drops of 5% red cell suspension to each tube and mix gently .

Centrifuge at 1500 rpm for 1 min only, or incubate at 37 °C for 30 min.

7.3.7.1 Observation

In the centrifuged tube, red cell sediment (button) will be seen at the bottom of the tube. Gently tap the bottom of the tube by a spring action of index finger and dislodge the button. Watch the behavior of the red cell button against a well-illuminated white background.

Observation

Red cells form one or more clumps with clear supernatant fluid	Positive
Red cells resuspend easily, without any visible clumping	Positive

Observation

Presence of small clumps	Positive
Hemolysis of red cells	Positive
Red cells resuspended easily without visible clumps	Negative

7.3.7.2 Confirmatory Test

Take a drop of suspension from the centrifuged tube with the help of micropipette on a microscopic slide, and confirm result under 100 × for type of agglutination as under (Table 7.6).

7.3.8 Reverse Serum Grouping by Tube Method

7.3.8.1 Procedure

Prepare three small tubes (10 × 75 mm) and label them as A, B, and O.

Prepare 5% red cell suspension of known A, B, and group O in separate tubes and label them separately.

Add two drops of 5% known red cell suspension in tube A.

Add two drops of known B group suspension in tube B.

Add two drops of known O red cell suspension in tube O.

Add two drops of serum to be tested in tubes, labeled as A and B.

Centrifuge all the three test tubes at 1500 rpm for 1 min, or incubate at room temperature for 1 h.

Examine the hemagglutination reaction against well-illuminated white background at eye level.

If hemagglutination is not visible, or there is weak reaction, resuspend the cells gently, and incubate at room temperature for 15 min, and then centrifuge at 1500 rpm for 1 min only, and see the result.

Table 7.6 Grading of agglutination

Large clumps with clear background	Clear agglutination
Smaller clumps with some free cells in the field	Weak agglutination
All red cells are free	No agglutination

Always use serum (instead of plasma) for reverse grouping as plasma may lead to non-detection of weak or complement-binding antibodies.

7.3.8.2 Advantages of Tube Method

Reverse grouping is more marked in tube method in comparison with the slide method, hence the method of choice.

It is more sensitive than the slide method.

It allows for fairly long incubation without drying up of the tubes' contents. Centrifugation involved enhances the reaction allowing weaker antigens and antibodies to be detected.

The method is simple and the results are reproducible.

The method is clean and more hygienic and requires small amount of reagent and test sample (Table 7.7).

7.3.9 Sources of Errors in ABO Grouping

Errors during ABO blood grouping usually present as discrepancies in the cell and serum grouping. The important factors leading to such problems could be due to (Table 7.8):

- **Factors related to red cells**
- **Factor related to serum**

Serum from persons with agammaglobulinemia may not contain detectable ABO antibodies.

The reactivity of reagent and red blood cells may diminish over the dating period.

Aged samples, subgroups, cold agglutinins, some diseased states, or patient age may impair test results.

Weak or missing reaction in reverse typing: It may be due to a decreased titer of antibody in the serum or plasma. The titer may be affected by age of sample, age of the patient, or certain

Table 7.7 Showing matched results of forward and reverse grouping

Cell grouping		Serum grouping		Interpretation		
Anti-A	Anti-B	A cells	B cells	Cell group	Serum group	Confirmed
Positive	Negative	Negative	Positive	A	A	A
Positive	Negative	Positive	Positive	A	O	A_2
Negative	Positive	Positive	Negative	B	B	B
Positive	Positive	Negative	Negative	AB	AB	AB
Positive	Positive	Positive	Negative	AB	B	A_2 B
Negative	Negative	Positive	Positive	O	O	O

Table 7.8 Sources of errors in ABO grouping

False positive	False negative
Drying of the slide	Inactive serum sample
Use of infected sera	No addition of the serum in test tube
Contaminated test sample	Contaminated red cells
Presence of unexpected antibodies	Outdated or contaminated antisera
Rouleaux formation	Defective technical procedure

diseased states. If the titer is too low, agglutination after centrifugation may be decreased.

If an expected agglutination is not present (or very weak): Either allow the tubes to stand 15–30 min at room temperature or in the refrigerator for 10–15 min. Resuspend the tubes, spin, and read and record results of 4 °C reaction. At this point the reverse type should be correct if the titer was weakened.

7.3.10 Cold Agglutinin (Anti-M and Anti-P1)

If the patient's antibody screen demonstrates a cold agglutinin, the serum/plasma and cells for the reverse typing may need to be prewarmed prior to adding the two together.

In such cases prewarm serum/plasma and cells separately for 10 min, and then the procedure is performed.

For a strong cold agglutinin: The patient's cells may need to be washed with prewarmed saline and typing reagents incubated for the forward type.

7.3.11 Quality Control

To recognize reagent deterioration, the reactivity of all blood grouping reagents should be confirmed on each day of use by testing known positive and negative controls.

7.3.12 How to Differentiate Between Rouleaux Formation and True Agglutination

The rouleaux formation is due to the presence of increased globulin; an example is multiple myeloma. In this, the red cells, as seen under the microscope, like stacks of coins. In rouleaux formation, the red cells will disperse, when a drop of saline is added on the microscopic slide. In true agglutination the cells will not disperse.

Infected blood cell sample will agglutinate spontaneously.

7.3.13 Causes of Variable Reaction

Most common is defective test procedure by inexperienced technician. The centrifugal force applied to form a red cell button should not be more than 1500 rpm for 1 min only. Over-centrifugation causes the red cells to adhere to the bottom of the test tube so that vigorous agitation is necessary for resuspension of red cells. During such vigorous agitation, weak agglutination may be dispersed causing false negative reaction.

7.3.14 Grouping of Cord Blood of Infant

Wash cord red cells five times with large volume (8 mL) of normal saline to minimize errors due to Wharton's jelly. Reactions in cell grouping may be weak as ABO antigens are not fully developed at birth and corresponding ABO antibodies are usually absent; therefore, only cell grouping is recommended till 6 months of age.

7.3.15 Microplate Technique Method for ABO Grouping

Microwell plate consists of a small polystyrene plate with 96 small wells, each of which can hold about 200–300 μm of reagent. There are three types of microplates, U-type, V-type, and flat-type well. U-type well is generally used in blood bank as it is easier to read the results in U-bottom plates. The principle is same as for agglutination in tube method. 200 μm of red cell suspension and same amount antisera are added to the microtiter plate wells, followed by centrifugation of the microtiter plate at 200 g for 1 min after 15 min of incubation.

- **Positive result**: carpet of red cells which line the bottom of the well
- **Negative result**: compact button with smooth edges which streams when the plate is tilted

7.3.15.1 Advantages of Microplate ABO Grouping

The method requires small volume of test sera, making it cost-effective.

It provides easy handling of a microplate and fast results.

Batching of samples can be achieved with considerable economy in space and time.

The test time is further reduced in well-equipped laboratories having microplate hardware items, e.g., reagent dispenser, sample handler, and cell washer.

Large batches of plates can be predispensed with antisera and reagent red cells before testing.

The technique of microplate grouping may be automated by on-line data capture in larger laboratories, which may help in:

(a) Reduction in reading and transcription errors
(b) Saving test time
(c) Use of bar codes for samples and microplate identification
(d) Integration into a comprehensive computer system for storage of data

7.3.16 Column or Gel Agglutination Method for ABO Grouping

This technology is straightforward, sensitive, and relatively easy to operate for laboratory technician. Here, the column is made of small microtubes that contains dextran acrylamide gel (which functions as a reaction medium and a size filter) matrix to trap agglutinates. Serum or red cells are mixed with anti-A, anti-B, and anti-D reagents in microtubes under controlled incubation and centrifugation. The gel particles trap the agglutinates, whereas non-agglutinated blood cells are allowed to pass through the column. The analysis time can be reduced by using glass beads in place of gel material, since in this way, faster centrifugation speeds can be achieved, which leads to rapid results.

7.3.16.1 Interpretation

- **Positive**: agglutinated cells forming a red cell line on the surface of gel or agglutinates dispersed in gel
- **Negative**: compact button of cells on the bottom of the microtube

7.3.16.2 Advantages of Microplate ABO Grouping

The method requires small volume of test sera, making it cost-effective.

This provides easy handling of a microplate and fast results.

Batching of samples can be achieved with considerable economy in space and time.

The test time is further reduced in well-equipped laboratories having microplate hardware items, e.g., reagent dispenser, sample handler, and cell washer.

Large batches of plates can be predispensed with antisera and reagent red cells before testing.

The technique of microplate grouping may be automated by on-line data capture in larger laboratories, which may help in:

(a) Reduction in reading and transcription errors
(b) Saving test time
(c) Use of bar codes for samples and microplate identification
(d) Integration into a comprehensive computer system for storage of data

Solid Phase Red Cell Adherence Assay (SPRCA): It in place of this is one of the two newly developed tubeless methods to improve sensitivity and specificity in ABO grouping, Rh phenotyping, and Kell determination. This method have gained wide acceptance following successful adaptation to fully automated platforms. The method uses a polystyrene microplate in which wells are coated with reagent red cells or red cell stroma.

In indirect test, serum sample is added, and if antibodies are present, they are captured by the antigen on the coated red cells. Indicator red cells which are coated with monoclonal IgG are added, and the mixture is centrifuged. Indicator red cells are attached to the antibody that was captured by coated red cells.

Positive reactions are indicated by the adherence of red blood cells over the entire surface of the wells.

Negative reactions form discrete red blood cell buttons in the center of the wells. The uniformity of the reaction patterns permits an objective reading of the results, both visually and spectrophotometrically.

Advantage

- Detecting A and B subgroups and D variants, the solid phase method was found to be more sensitive when compared with the agglutination method.
- Due to the ease of handling of the new solid phase assay and the unequivocal test results, the method is suitable for manual routine testing in small- to medium-sized laboratories as well as for automation.
- The reaction patterns can easily be interpreted visually or by computer software-supported readers. Resultant microplates can be stored in a refrigerator for 3 weeks.

7.3.17 Testing for A_1 and A_2 Subgroups

Anti-A_1 reagent is used to differentiate A_1 and A_2 subgroups. Source of anti-A reagent is lectin—Dolichos biflorus.

Human anti-A_1 (by adsorption of group B anti-A serum by A_2 cells) Dolichos biflorus lectin reacts specifically with A_1 antigen and causes agglutination. It is stored at 4–8 °C and may be frozen at −20 °C for prolonged storage.

7.3.17.1 Procedure

Add one drop of anti-A_1 into a clean, dry test tube.

Add one drop of 5% saline suspension of patient's cells.

Mix and leave at RT for 5–10 min.

The results can be read immediately after 1 min.

Gently agitate and examine for agglutination.

Interpretation: Presence of agglutination indicates A_1 blood group.

Controls: Perform the test using known A_1 cells and A_2 cells.

In routine laboratory procedures, ABO and Rh (D) grouping is usually performed in parallel.

Anti-D sera are of three types:

Anti-D IgM
Anti-D IgG
Anti-D blend of IgM monoclonal + IgG polyclonal

Anti-D serum (IgG) for saline or rapid tube test (high-protein medium) contains macromolecular additives, and results are highly reproducible.

Polyclonal anti-D sera available for slide and rapid tube test are usually unsuitable for microplate use. Usually a dilution of 1:20 of ABO antisera and 1:10 of anti-D antisera gives good results.

7.3.18 Controls for Rh (D) Grouping

Known O Rh (D)-positive and O Rh (D)-negative cells may be used as controls with monoclonal anti-D reagent.

7.3.19 Rh (D) Grouping

In all the blood transfusion laboratories, Rh (D) grouping is performed along with the ABO grouping and same techniques, as used for ABO grouping may also be employed for Rh typing.

Methods for Rh (D) Grouping
Slide method
Tube method
Microplate method

7.3.19.1 Rh (D) Grouping by Slide Method

Perform the test with 40–50% red cell suspension or whole blood.

On a prewarm glass slide (40 °C), place two drops of red cell suspension in the center of the slide.

Add two drops of anti-D serum on the drop of blood.

Mix the red cells with serum by toothpick or by the corner of another glass slide.

Tilt the slide back and forth and observe for agglutination which is recognized by the clumping of the red cells.

Do not observe longer than 2 min.

A positive and negative control test must be run each day to obtain reliable result.

Slide method is less sensitive than the tube method, but it is easy to perform and gives reliable results in 99% of cases, hence the method of first choice in all routine testing.

7.3.19.2 Rh (D) Grouping by Tube Method

Perform the test with 5% red cell suspension.

Place four glass tubes of 10 × 75 mm on a rack, and label them as "T" for test sample, "P" for known Rh (D)-positive control, "N" for known negative control, and "SA" for serum albumin control.

Add one drop of anti-Rh sera into the first three tubes marked as "T," "P," and "N." Add one drop of bovine albumin 22 % in tube marked as "SA."

Add two drops of red cell suspension tube marked as "T" and "SA."

Add two drops of known Rh-positive red cell suspension in tube "P."

Add two drops of known Rh-negative red cell suspension in tube "N."

Incubate all the tubes at 37 °C for 30 min or centrifuge all the tubes at 1500 rpm for 1 min.

Examine the agglutination reaction in each tube by dislodging the button gently.

Agglutination will be recognized by the formation of small clumps in a clear liquid.

Tap the bottom of the tube, clumps whirl up and then settle down. It denotes positive reaction and the cells are identified as Rh (+) positive.

If the red cells resuspend homogenously with no visible clumps, they are identified as Rh-negative (−) cells (Table 7.9).

7.3.19.3 Sources of Errors in Rh (D) Grouping and Resolving Rh Problems

Inaccurate or incorrect results in Rh grouping may occur due to technical errors. These can result from defects in equipment, reagents, specimen, and techniques or through wrong interpretation.

Improper identification of test sample and mixing of samples is of common occurrence leading to administration of wrong blood to wrong patient.

Always perform the test with known positive and negative controls on each day.

Follow the manufacture instructions precisely during test performance.

In case of discrepant test result, obtain a fresh sample of blood, and repeat the test with known positive and negative controls. Contaminated,

Table 7.9 Interpretation of the test

	Tube T	Tube P	Tube N	Tube SA	Interpretation
Agglutination	Positive	Positive	Negative	Negative	Rh positive
	Negative	Positive	Negative	Negative	Rh negative
	Positive	Negative	Negative	Negative	Invalid
	Negative	Negative	Negative	Negative	Invalid

Tube labeled as "P" should show agglutination
Tube labeled as "N" shows absent agglutination
Tube labeled as "SA" should show lack of agglutination

old, hemolyzed sample may produce unreliable results.

Heavy red cell suspension in tube method, light red cell suspension in slide method, over-centrifugation, drying of the slides during hot weather, or observation of slide beyond the 2 min period may lead to improper results. Failure to recognize hemolysis can give false negative results.

Coating of the red cells with autoantibody may produce a false positive result. In such cases perform tube method with washed red cells.

Rouleaux formation can produce false positive result in slide method. To resolve this add few drops of warm saline and observe the finding.

Thomsen phenomenon: Bacterial contamination of the blood sample can lead to iso-agglutinability and produce panagglutination (Hübener–Friedenreich–Thomsen phenomenon; T agglutination; polyagglutination). Obtain a fresh sample and repeat the test.

Check the bacterial contamination of anti-D—it is recognized by cloudiness of the reagent—and loss of activity is seen from absence of agglutination in known Rh-positive control red cells.

The causes of weak agglutination reaction are weak anti-D sera and red cells that belong to Du.

Presence of cold agglutinins (antibodies) in the test serum can cause autoagglutination. It is most commonly seen in blood group Ii, MNS, and P group. High titer of cold antibodies is a constant feature of *Mycoplasma* infection.

To resolve this warm the reagent and red cell suspension at 37 °C, and then perform the test procedure. Immunological reaction due to cold agglutinins disappears at body temperature (37 °C).

7.3.19.4 Saline Agglutination Test for Rh

Prepare 5% washed red cell suspension of test sample.

Take anti-D from two different manufacturer brand company to assess the potency of test reagent and producibility of the test result.

Place one drop of anti-D from one brand in cleaned tube labeled D_1, and place one drop of anti-D from a different manufacturer in a clean tube labeled D_2.

Place one drop of bovine albumin 22%/control reagent in another tube labeled C.

Add 1 drop of 5% test cell suspension to each tube.

Mix it well and centrifuge at 1000 rpm for 1 min (in case of using IgG anti-D, incubate at 37 °C for 10 min, and centrifuge (spin tube method), or incubate at 37 °C for 60 min (sedimentation method)). Resuspend the cell button and look for agglutination. All negative results must be confirmed under microscope (Table 7.10).

Albumin increases the dielectric constant of the medium and thus reduces the zeta potential. Due to this effect, the electrical repulsion between the red blood cells is less and the cells agglutinate. Mostly bovine albumin 22% is used, as higher concentrations can cause rouleaux formation.

- **Positive test**: Agglutination in anti-D (both tubes) and smooth suspension in control tube
- **Negative test**: Smooth suspension in all the tubes (test and control)

Table 7.10 Interpretation of the test result of the

	Tube D_1	Tube D_2	Tube C	Interpretation
Agglutination	Positive	Positive	Negative	Rh positive
	Negative	Negative	Negative	Rh negative
	Positive	Positive	Positive	Invalid test

Table 7.11 Comparison of ABO and Rh grouping methods

Parameter	ABO grouping	Rh grouping
Blood group	A, B, AB, and O	Rh positive and negative
Forward grouping	Yes	Yes
Reverse grouping	Yes	No
Antisera	IgM	IgG or IgM
Reaction temperature	Room temperature	37 °C or at room temperature
Enhancer requirement	No	Yes

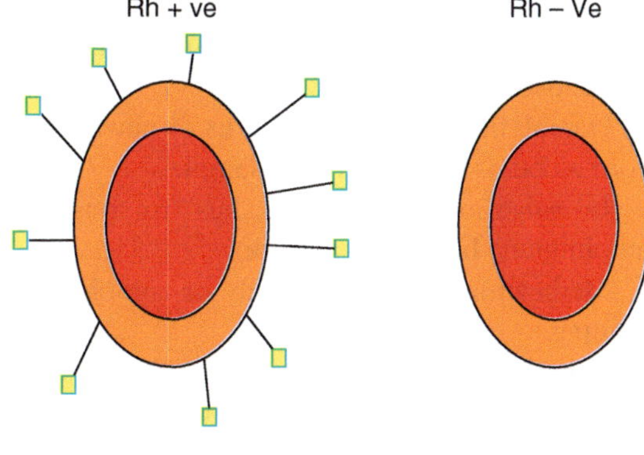

Fig. 7.2 Rh antigens

Test is considered invalid if both test and control tubes show a positive reaction.

In discrepant results, obtain a fresh sample of patient blood and repeat the test (Table 7.11 and Fig. 7.2).

Rh (D) grouping by microplate method: **It** is a polystyrene plate consisting of 96 microwells of either U or V shape. Grouping is carried out in microwells. This method is sensitive and ideal for large number of samples.

Antihuman globulin (AGT) or Coombs test: It in place of this was first developed by **Robin Coombs,** British immunologist, in 1945. The Coombs test is used to detect antibodies that act against the surface of the red blood cells.

There are two types of antihuman globulin test—direct and indirect.

- **Direct antihuman globulin test** (DAT): The test recognizes the sensitized red cells which occur within the body in cases of hemolytic reaction of the newborn and autoimmune hemolytic anemia.
- **Indirect antihuman globulin test (IAT)**: It in place of this is used to detect sensitization of red cells which is done in the laboratory (in vitro). It recognizes sensitized red cells when the by incubating the red cells with the corresponding antibody at 37 °C for 30 min. The indirect Coombs test is used only in prenatal testing of pregnant women and in testing blood prior to a transfusion.

7.3.20 Reagent Used for Coombs Test

Antihuman serum (Coombs antisera) is used in determining the presence or absence of red blood cell antibody or components of human complement on red blood cells. Accordingly antihuman serum is used for compatibility testing, antibody detection, antibody identification, testing for the variant of the Rho (D) antigen (DU tests), and umbilical cord red blood cell testing. Antihuman serum may be used in the direct antiglobulin test and in the indirect antiglobulin test to detect antibodies and/or complement on red blood cells.

Bovine albumin is primarily used to enhance the reactivity of blood grouping antibodies, either in direct agglutination tests or indirect antiglobulin test which can be qualitatively used in antibody detection, identification, titration, and control of Rh typing.

7.3.20.1 Direct Coombs (Antiglobulin Test) (DAT)

The test detects antibodies bound to erythrocytes in vivo.

Indications of the DAT

Investigation of the hemolytic transfusion reactions whether it is acute or chronic. It requires posttransfusion blood sample.

Hemolytic disease of the fetus or newborn—cord blood or newborn blood sample.

Investigation of autoantibodies (for possible autoimmune hemolytic anemia).

Medication-induced antibody or complement binding.

Sample required: EDTA blood of the patient is necessary to chelate calcium (a necessary component of C3 activation) so that in vitro C3 fixation will not occur.

This test is performed to detect the anti-D antibody or any other antibodies to the red cell surface within the blood stream. This occurs in the following conditions:

When there is an Rh-positive baby in the womb of a sensitized Rh-negative woman, the antibodies produced in the mother's serum cross the placenta, and after entering the baby's blood stream, these antibodies will attach to the baby's Rh-positive red cells. These coated and sensitized cells are clumped and removed from the circulation, causing hemolytic anemia also known as hemolytic disease of the newborn or erythroblastosis fetalis. When the baby is born, the baby's cord blood is collected from the umbilical cord and tested to detect anti-D antibodies coated on red cells (Box 7.2).

Box 7.2 Causes of Positive Direct Coombs (Antiglobulin) Test

Erythroblastosis fetalis
Most cases of autoimmune hemolytic anemia
Delayed hemolytic transfusion reaction
Drug-induced: methyldopa red cell sensitization
Test is positive in healthy blood donors 1:8000

Procedure

Wash the red cells of the test sample four times with 8 mL of normal saline to remove free globulin.

Decant completely at the end of the last washing.

The last wash should always have a clear supernatant with no signs of hemolysis.

Take a glass tube of 10 × 75 mm and label as "T."

Transfer two drops of 5% washed red cells in tube T.

Add two drops of antihuman globulin serum to the tube T.

Mix well and centrifuge at 1500 rpm for 1 min.

Examine for agglutination by holding against illuminated white surface and tapping the bottom of the tube. Hold the tube at an angle, shake well until all the cells are dislodged, and then tilt the tube gently, back and forth, until even suspension of cells or agglutinates is observed.

If no agglutination is seen, leave the tube at room temperature for 10 min, and then recentrifuge at 1500 rpm for 1 min. A weaker reactive antibody will show delayed reaction. This is positive test (Table 7.12).

7.3.20.2 Indirect Antiglobulin (Coombs) Test

Here the sensitization of red cells is done in the laboratory (in vitro) by incubating the red cells

Table 7.12 Application of direct antiglobulin test (DAT) in immunohematology

Clinical course	Caused by	Source of IgG
Transfusion reaction	Donor red cells coated with IgG	Patient antibody
HDNB	Fetal red cells coated with IgG	Maternal antibody crossing the placenta
AIHA	IgG or C3 on patient's red cells	Patient's autoantibody
Drug-related mechanism	IgG–drug complex attached to red cells	Immune complex formed with drugs

with the corresponding antibody from patient serum at 37 °C for 30 min.

An indirect Coombs 10s test can be used to determine whether there are antibodies to the Rh factor in the mother's blood. In this case a normal (negative) result indicates that the mother has not developed antibodies against the fetus's blood and that the fetus is not presently in danger from problems relating to Rh incompatibility.

An abnormal (positive) indicates that the mother has developed antibodies to the fetal red blood cells and is sensitized and an Rh-positive fetus has a possibility of having hemolytic disease of the newborn. A positive test cannot indicate the amount of fetal harm that has occurred or is likely to occur. If test results show that antibody amounts are increasing during pregnancy, the fetus may be at greater risk of harm.

Rh negative will not be affected, even if the mother is sensitized.

Indications

This test is performed to detect the presence of Rh antibodies or other antibodies in patient's serum in case of the following:

Whether an Rh-negative woman married to an Rh-positive husband has developed anti-Rh antibodies in her blood.

Anti-D may be produced in the blood of any Rh-negative person by previous exposure to D antigen by (A) transfusion of Rh-positive blood, (B) pregnancy if the infant is Rh positive, (C) abortion of Rh-positive fetus, (D) any vaginal instrumentation, (€) stillborn fetus, and (F) accidental contamination with Rh-positive blood by any injury.

Crossmatching for blood transfusion.

Detection and identification of antibody: specific antibody—usually isoimmunization from previous transfusion.

Non-specific autoantibody in acquired hemolytic anemia.

RBC phenotyping in genetic and forensic medicine.

Identification of syngeneic twins for bone marrow transplantation.

Sample required: Serum sample of the patient.

Procedure

Label the three glass tubes of 10 × 75 mm as "**T**" (test serum), as "**PC**" (positive control), and as "**NC**" (negative control).

Add two drops of test serum in the tube labeled as T.

Add one drop of anti-D in the tube labeled as PC.

Add one drop of saline in the tube labeled as NC.

Add two drops of 5% red cell saline suspension of pooled O Rh (D)-positive cells in all three tubes.

Incubate all the tubes in water bath at 37 °C for 30 min.

Remove all the tubes from water bath and wash four times with 4 mL of saline to remove excess serum with no free antibodies. Decant completely after the last washing.

Add two drops of Coombs serum (antihuman serum) to all three tubes and mix well.

Keep it at room temperature for 5 min.

Centrifuge all the tubes at 1500 rpm for 1 min.

Resuspend the cells and examine for hemagglutination macroscopically and microscopically for (Tables 7.13 and 7.14).

Causes of false negative indirect antiglobulin test (IAT) are:

- Failure to wash RBCs adequately.
- Improper procedure: failure to add antiglobulin reagents, delay in adding AHG. reagent, or expired AHG reagent.
- Too little serum added/too much reagent RBCs added.
- Undercentrifugation.
- Improper incubation temperature or time.

Table 7.13 Interpretation

Tubes	Observation	Conclusions
PC	Agglutination positive	Correctly performed test procedure
	No agglutination	Defective Coombs serum—repeat the test
NC	No agglutination, since saline does not contain anti-D	
T	Agglutination positive	Patient's serum contains anti-D
T	No agglutination	Patient's serum does not contain anti-D

Table 7.14 Application of indirect antiglobulin test in immunohematology

Procedure	Purpose
Antibody screening	Detects antibodies with specificity to red cell antigen
Antibody identification	Identifies specificity of red cell antibodies
Crossmatch	Determines serological compatibility between donor and patient before transfusion
Antigen typing	Identifies a specific red cell antigen in a patient or donor

- Improper serum and cell ratio.
- Misinterpretation in testing: weak positive can be misinterpreted as negative; for confirmation use microscope for better observation.

Causes of false positive indirect antiglobulin test (IAT) are as follows:

- Specimen collected in 5–10% dextrose IV line (dextrose causes in vitro complement fixation).
- Patient is septic or specimen is contaminated by bacteria (T activation causing panagglutination).
- Sensitized patient RBCs (positive DAT with allo- or autoantibodies).
- Contamination of saline with materials that can cause spontaneous aggregation of RBCs (e.g., colloidal silica from glass bottles) or dirty glassware.
- Improper procedure: over-centrifugation.
- Over-incubation with enzyme-treated cells.
- Improper AHG reagent.
- Potent agglutinins such as strong cold agglutinins.
- Improper use of enhancement reagents (Tables 7.15 and 7.16).

Table 7.15 Differences between direct and indirect antiglobulin test

Direct antiglobulin test (DAT)	Indirect antiglobulin test (IAT)
Detect IgG and complement-coated red cells	Detect IgG and complement-coated red cells
IgG attached to red cells has occurred within the patient's body	IgG attachment to red cells occurred during the incubation phase outside body
One-stage procedure	Two-stage procedure
Patient's red cells are treated with AHG without an incubation step	Test requires an incubation step before addition of AHG
Test indicated for HDNB, AIHA, and transfusion reaction	Used as a reaction phase in different immunological test

Table 7.16 Compatibility testing

Problem	Causes	Resolution
ABO phenotype error	Error in patient's identification	Repeat ABO
	Sample error	Redraw pt. sample
Unexpected antibodies	Cold alloantibody M, P1	Test panel cells
	Anti-A1 in A2	Test A2 cells
	Cold autoantibody (I, IH)	Determine clinical significant antibody

7.3.21 Weak Expression of the Rh D Antigen (Du)

The term Du is widely used to describe cells which have a quantitative reduction in the expression of their RhD antigen or qualitative variation in RhD antigen expression; these are referred to as partial D. Weak D individuals may also be partial D. There are four D phenotypes (D+, D−, weak D, partial D).

Weak D testing is done on all prenatal patients and candidates for Rh immunoglobulin. Weak D testing is also done on Rh-negative donors to ensure they are truly D negative.

Indirect Coombs is applied in Du testing: Du factor is a variant D antigen present on the red cells of individuals of Du blood type. Red cells carrying Du factor can falsely be considered as Rh negative if of Du test is not performed. The Du reacts with anti-D but does not cause hemagglutination due to the fact that reaction is not so strong enough to be visualized. In this the red cells are sensitized and are coated with anti-D (IgG) following incubation. Following repeated washing of red cells with normal saline, Du is recognized by reacting with AHG.

Table 7.17 Interpretation of the test result

Observation	Anti-D serum (T)	Bovine albumin (C)	Interpretation
1	No agglutination	No agglutination	Du negative
2	Agglutination+	No agglutination	Du positive
3	Agglutination+	Agglutination+	Test invalid

7.3.21.1 Principle

Red cells that react weakly or not at all in direct agglutination test (DAT) with anti-D may react with anti-D by the indirect antiglobulin test (IAT). Red cells that fail to react 2+ in direct agglutination tests with anti-D are incubated with anti-D at 37 °C and examined for agglutination. The red cells are washed to remove unbound antibody (IgG anti-D) and then tested with anti-IgG.

7.3.21.2 Du Testing

Prepare a 5% suspension of red cells in saline.

Take two 10 × 75 mm glass tube and label them as "**T**" for serum and "**C**" for albumin.

Add two drops of 5% red cell suspension in both the tube marked as "T" and "C."

Add one drop of anti-D serum to the tube marked as "T."

Add one drop of bovine albumin 22% in the tube marked as "C."

Place both the tubes in water bath at 37 °C for 30 min.

Wash both the tubes with 4 mL of normal saline three times with repeated centrifugation at 1500 rpm.

Decant both the tubes after last washing.

Add two drops of antihuman globulin (containing anti-IgG) to the sedimented cells, dislodge the button, and mix the cells gently with antiserum.

Centrifuge both the tubes at 1500 rpm for 1 min.

Resuspend the cells by gentle agitation, and examine agglutination macroscopically, and confirm the result microscopically.

7.3.21.3 Observation

Tests should be read immediately after centrifugation. Delay may cause bound IgG to dissociate from red cells and either leave too little IgG to detect or neutralize AHG reagent causing false negative results (Table 7.17).

A true weak D should give at least a 2+ positive result. Weaker results may be due to mixed field agglutination in an Rh-negative individual who received Rh-positive blood, or vice versa. Obtain a recent transfusion history in patients who give inconclusive weak D results.

Slide Technique for **Antigen (Du)**.

Take a clean glass slide and label each half as M and G.

Add one drop of IgM on glass slide marked as M.

Add one drop of IgG glass slide marked as G.

Add one drop of the test 5% red cell suspension on both the portion of the slide.

Mix well by gently and continuously rocking the slide for 30 s, and incubate the slide for 5 min at room temperature, with mixing to and fro.

Examine macroscopically for agglutination at the end of 5 min and record the results.

7.4 Compatibility Testing or Crossmatching

The final criteria of whether donor blood is safe to a patient depends on ABO and Rh grouping and running of compatibility test to see any signs of compatibility or incompatibility. Under most circumstances, if grouping and Rh typing tests have been performed accurately and if the donor blood of the same group and Rh type has been selected for testing and transfusion, they will be found to be compatible. However, there are occasions when the donor may have antibodies in his serum or the patient may have antibodies in his serum. There may have been a mistake in performing, reading, or recording the blood grouping and Rh typing results. Considering all these possibilities, a compatibility test is essential before all transfusions. The procedure used to determine compatibility of donor and recipient's blood is called the crossmatch.

Purpose: to find out compatibility of donor's red cells with patient's serum in order to avoid transfusion reactions. This procedure is performed in two parts:

- **Major crossmatch**: In this crossmatch the donor red cells are mixed with patient's serum.
- **Minor crossmatch**: In this crossmatch the patient's red cells are mixed with donor's serum.

Collect 2 mL of the recipient's fresh blood, while donor's blood is obtained from the pilot tube. The donor's blood from the pilot tube should not be more than 21 days and be constantly stored at 4 °C.

Principle: Serum of the recipient is tested against the red cells of the donor under different conditions in order to establish their compatibility or non-agglutination. Agglutination in any of the conditions indicates the presence of incompatible antibody in patient. The antibody can be natural or immune.

There are three phases of compatibility testing as described below.

- **Saline phase**: In this phase the immunologic reaction between red cells suspended in saline and the antibody occurs at room temperature.
- **Thermophase**: In this phase the red cells are suspended in serum which contains the antibody with bovine albumin 22% (protein) and incubated for 30 min at 37 °C.
- **Antihuman globulin (AHG) phase**: In this phase the incubated red cells are washed (to remove free globulin) and reacted with antihuman globulin serum (Coombs serum).

ABO incompatibility is recognized in the saline phase by the presence of agglutination.

The presence of agglutination in other phases indicates the presence of immune, incomplete, or irregular antibodies.

No agglutination in any of the three phases indicates compatible donor's and recipient's blood.

7.4.1 Preparation of Donor Red Cells for Crossmatching

ACD anticoagulated donor's blood should not be more than 21 days old. Collect the donor blood from the pilot tube on blood bag, and confirm ABO and Rh (D) group by slide method. After confirming the blood group, donor red cells are taken out of the clot and washed four times with 4 mL of saline with repeated centrifugation. After the last wash, prepare 5% red cell suspension. Add 0.1 mL of packed washed red cells in 1.9 mL of normal saline. It will give 5% red cell suspension.

7.4.2 Preparation of Patient Red Cells for Crossmatching

Collect the recipient's blood freshly, and confirm ABO and Rh (D) group by slide method, and prepare 5% red cell suspension as described above.

7.4.2.1 Procedure

Take two small glass tubes of 10 × 75 mm and label them as tube 1 and 2.

In tube 1 add two drops of patient's serum and two drops of donor's 5% red cell suspension (major crossmatch).

In tube 2 add two drops of donor serum and two drops of patient's 5% red cell suspension (minor crossmatch).

Mix and centrifuge at 1500 rpm for 1 min.

Gently dislodge the red cell button, and examine for agglutination and hemolysis macroscopically and microscopically.

If both tubes 1 and 2 do not show agglutination, the blood is compatible. If any of the tube shows agglutination, the blood is incompatible.

7.4.3 Sources of Errors in Crossmatching

Rouleaux formation: In this condition the red cells show characteristic roll of coins under the microscope, and this is due to high concentration of globulin in conditions like multiple myeloma or previous administration of plasma expander like dextran.

Remedy: Add one drop of normal saline on the slide; if it disappears, it is due to rouleaux; if it does not disperse, then it is due to hemagglutination.

Panagglutination reactions: Occasionally here donor cells will agglutinate with any or some sera. It is usually due to infected red cells. If positive, do not transfuse donor's blood.

Cold agglutination: In this process hemagglutination reaction usually appears below 18 °C and disappears at 37 °C. It is due to autoagglutination. Presence of cold agglutinin in patient's serum is usually ignored and donor blood can be transfused.

Cord red cells: can result false positive result due to the presence of Wharton's jelly.

Solution: Wash the fetal red cells thoroughly with large volume (8 mL) of saline six times before testing.

Autoantibody: The presence of autoantibodies may cause agglutination of the patient's own red cells. Autoantibodies are produced in cases of hemolytic anemias, and they are directed toward the patient's own red cells. Presence of autoantibody gives positive DAT.

Solution: Ascertain the cause of autoagglutination. Wash the red cells four times with 4 mL of normal saline, elute in warm saline, and then perform the crossmatch. It will resolve the problem.

7.4.4 False Negative Reactions

Causes are inactive serum or no addition of serum during the test procedure.

Solution: Run positive and negative control each day.

Set the test in duplicate when the need arises.

7.4.5 Emergency Crossmatch Procedure

Dire emergency with no lead time: Use and supply O Rh (D)-negative blood without crossmatching.

Lead time of 15–30 min: Perform ABO and Rh (D) grouping and choose group-specific blood.

Lead time of 30–45 min: Perform ABO and Rh grouping and quick crossmatch.

Lead time of more than 45 min: Go through routine procedure.

7.5 Compatibility Report

Date:
Blood bank laboratory reference number:
Patient's name Age Sex
Patient's blood group Rh group
Donor blood group Rh group
Donor blood sample (bag number) is found to be compatible with blood sample (blood bank laboratory reference number).
Supplied on at
Blood sample supplied was tested for HIV 1 and 2, hepatitis B, hepatitis C, and VDRL
Signature of resident doctor
Name of resident doctor

7.6 Antibody Screening Test

The antibody screening test is performed to detect the presence of unexpected antibodies, especially alloantibodies in the serum to antigens of the non-ABO blood group system: Duffy, Kell, Kidd, MNS, P, and certain Rh types that are considered clinically significant. Naturally occurring anti-A and anti-B are the only RBC antibodies in normal human serum or plasma. All others are unexpected and can be divided into alloantibodies (an antibody to an antigen that an individual lacks) and autoantibodies (an antibody to an antigen a person has). The development of alloantibodies can significantly complicate transfusion therapy and results in difficulties in crossmatching of blood.

Investigation of immune-mediated hemolytic anemia.

Identifying antibody(ies) in prenatal patients to assist in determining the risk for hemolytic disease of the fetus and newborn (HDFN).

In case of incompatible crossmatch or in the investigation of transfusion reaction, a search for the presence of atypical antibodies is required.

The antibody screening is routinely indicated in obstetric patient in whom detection and identification of the antibody, prior to delivery, allows adequate time for preparation to be made for the possible transfusion in the newborn infant.

Principle: Antibody screening is based on the indirect antihuman globulin or AHG test. Reagent O cells are subjected to all the phases of crossmatching. Presence of unexpected antibody will be recognized by the hemagglutination reaction or hemolysis of O cells. This usually occurs in thermophase (with protein) and AHG phase. The nature of the antibody is judged by the reaction phase. Absence of agglutination of red cells indicates that the patient's serum does not have unexpected antibodies.

Procedure: In a prelabeled test tube of 12 × 75 mm, collect 5 mL of patient's blood without any anticoagulant.

Allow it to stand for 30 min at room temperature.

Separate the serum in another tube and preserve it.

Prepare a 5% red cell suspension in saline which will be used as autocontrol.

Take three test tubes of 12 × 75 mm and label them as I, II, and autocontrol (C).

These represent O Rh-positive reagent cells of group I and group II (from two different donor red cells) and the autocontrol which will have the patient's own red cells.

Prepare a 5% red cell suspension of group I and II and patient's red cells and label them.

Take another set of three test tubes and label them as 1, 2, and 3 (autocontrol).

Add two drops of test serum in all the tubes—1, 2, and 3 (autocontrol).

Add one drop of 5% red cell suspension O-positive tube I in the first tube as marked 1. Add one drop of 5% red cell suspension of O-positive red cells of donor in tube 2.

Add 5% suspension of the patient's red cell suspension in tube 3 (autocontrol).

To all the three tubes, add two drops of 22% bovine albumin along the slide of the tube. Albumin is added to lower zeta potential so cells can agglutinate without Coombs step and may detect Rh antibodies.

Mix gently and incubate at 37 °C for 30 min. This phase is required since IgG clinically significant antibodies are warm-reacting antibodies.

Centrifuge at 1500 rpm for 1 min.

Now look for agglutination and hemolysis.

If the reaction is negative, wash the red cells three times with excess volume of saline to remove the free globulin.

Do not overdo this step or else the cell-bound antibody may be lost by elution. The common way to wash is to decant the saline as completely as possible between each washing and to resuspend the cells completely with each addition of new saline (3/4 full test tube) each time. Shake well the cell button and add the saline in forceful stream.

If there is no agglutination, check the antiglobulin phase with Coombs positive control cells.

Interpretation: Agglutination in any phase indicates the presence of unexpected antibody in the serum provided the autocontrol (autocontrol) does not show any hemagglutination, i.e., the patient's cells do not agglutinate by themselves when exposed to the patient's own serum due to the presence of autoantibody.

If agglutination is seen in any of the other tubes (2 and 3), it indicates the presence of unexpected alloantibody.

The autocontrol should not show agglutination.

The test is of great value, but it does have its limitation.

A negative test does not necessarily mean that the serum lacks unexpected antibodies. It is possible that the corresponding antigen is not present on the reagent cells selected. Since the reagent O cells are pooled from two different donors, the chances are few. If screening cells do not react with the serum antibody, it can be safely considered that the serum does not have any unusual antibody. If agglutination is seen, the next step is to identify the antibody that is causing agglutination.

7.6.1 Elution of Antibodies

Elution in cases of hemolytic disease of the newborn or hemolytic anemia the offending antibody is coated on the sensitized red cells. This is detected by direct antihuman globulin test. In such cases, elution techniques are used to remove the antibody from the red cells followed by subsequent identification in elute. This process involves raising the temperature of the sample to about 56 °C. Raising the temperature will cause the antibody–antigen complex to break apart, thus freeing the antibodies. Elution removes antibody molecules from the red cell membrane either by disrupting the antigen or changing conditions to favor dissociation of antibody from antigen. The sample is then tested with different blood types to see which blood type causes the antibodies from the dried blood sample to combine with the blood antigens.

7.6.1.1 Indications of Elution of Antibodies

Autoimmune hemolytic anemia (AIHA).

Diagnosis of ABO hemolytic disease of the newborn (HDN).

Identification of specificity when multiple antibodies exist in a patient's serum or plasma.

Phenotyping of red cells in patients with a positive DAT.

7.6.1.2 Procedure

Centrifuge 2 mL of EDTA-treated blood sample from which eluate is to be made with the positive DAT.

Transfer the supernatant serum or plasma to a separate, properly labeled tube.

Place 20 drops of the red cells in a properly labeled 12 × 75 mm tube.

Wash the cells eight (8) times with large volumes of saline. Remove the supernatant saline with a pipette.

Mix cells vigorously between washes by adding a small volume of saline and thumping the tube vigorously with finger or covering the tube with Parafilm and inverting the tube until all cells are resuspended off the bottom of the tube.

If cells are not completely resuspended between washes, antibody may be trapped in between the packed RBCs, and this will cause a false positive reaction in the last wash as well as the eluate, and the procedure will need to be repeated.

The final wash should be performed by adding volume of saline equal to the volume of washed packed red cells.

Centrifuge (1500 rpm) for 1 min, and separate the supernatant to test for the presence of residual free-floating antibody. If positive, repeat the wash until the negative result is obtained.

The supernatant of the last wash is finally tested in parallel with eluate. The supernatant acts as the negative control that demonstrates that residual antibody has been removed before eluate is prepared from the red cells.

Add an equal volume of saline to the washed packed red cells in the centrifuge tube.

Place the tubes at 56 °C for 10 min, agitating the tube constantly during this time with two applicator sticks.

Centrifuge in prewarmed cups at high speed (3400 rpm for 1 min).

Remove the hemoglobin-tinted supernatant fluid. This is eluate.

Immediately transfer the supernatant eluate into a clean test tube, and test in parallel with the final wash supernatant.

Test the eluate for the presence of antibody.

Use the lost saline wash as the negative control.

Eluate can be stored overnight at 4 °C or at −20 °C for long period.

7.7 Titration of Anti-D

Antibody titration (ABT) of anti-D is a semi-quantitative method used to detect the reactivity of antibodies present in the patient's plasma. Antibody titration is used prenatally to screen for risk of hemolytic disease of the fetus and newborn (HDFN) and hemolytic reactions or for assessment in solid organ or hematopoietic stem cell transplant. To assess risk for HDFN, if the mother has a clinically significant alloantibody, ABT is performed. When the antibody and the titer strength are identified, ABT is periodically performed throughout pregnancy, where the results of previous samples are compared with recent test to determine increase in titer strength. A rise in anti-D titer would need to be at least 2 dilution increase between the current specimen and the previous month could indicate the possibility of hemolytic disease of the newborn.

7.7.1 Other Indication of Antibody Titration

Antibody titration is also used for screening blood products, particularly platelets and plasma. To decrease the risk of hemolytic transfusion reactions due to passive anti-A/anti-B antibodies, the titer of group O products is determined, and those with high titers (typically 1:100) are labeled and used for group O individuals only.

ABT has a role in preventing graft rejection for ABO-incompatible solid organ transplants of the heart, liver, and lung as well as in delaying erythroid engraftment after hematopoietic progenitor cell transplants.

Principle: Antibody titration involves a serial dilution of the serum. Each dilution is tested against the corresponding antigen. It provides a semiquantitative measure of the amount of antibody in a serum. The highest serum dilution where the agglutination is observed is the titer. Antibody titration involves a serial dilution of the serum in saline and testing of each dilution against the corresponding red cell antigen. In case of anti-D titration, the chosen red cells carry D antigen (Rh positive). Titration scores provide a semiquantitative measure of the amount of antibody in a serum. Titrations are most frequently performed by preparing progressively double dilutions of the serum. In the course of twofold dilutions and subsequent testing of hemagglutination, a point will arrive when the antibody is too dilute to bring about the immunological reaction between the agglutinogen present on red cells and agglutinin (antibody) present in diluted serum. The highest serum dilution where the agglutination is observed is the titer. For example, if the dilution is 1:64 (1 part of serum in 64 parts of saline), the titer is reported as 64.

Specimen: Collect 4 mL of patient's blood in a plain test tube. Allow it to clot. Centrifuge the tube at 1500 rpm and separate the serum in the second tube. This serum is used for the test.

Collect 4 mL of Rh-positive blood, and after washing prepare 5% red cell suspension (Table 7.18).

Add 0.1 mL of saline from tube number 2 to 10.

Add 0.1 mL of test serum in tubes 1 and 2 and mix well.

Transfer 0.1 mL of contents from tube number 2 to tube number 3. Mix well.

Continue this procedure till tube number 10. It will give final dilution of 512.

Add two drops of bovine albumin 22% in all the ten tubes. Mix well.

Table 7.18 Procedure: take 75 × 100 glass tubes without rims and label the tubes as follows

Tube	1	2	3	4	5	6	7	8	9	10
Dilution	1	2	4	8	16	32	64	128	256	512

Table 7.19 Showing antibody titer and score

Tube no.	1	2	3	4	5	6	7	8	9	10	Titer
Dilution	1	2	4	8	16	32	64	128	256	512	
Example 1	4+	4+	3+	3+	3+	2+	1+	0	0	0	64
Example 2	4+	4+	4+	4+	3+	2+	2+	1+	0	0	128
Example 3	3+	3+	2+	2+	1+	1+	0	0	0	0	32
Example 4	0	0	0	1+	1	2+	3+	3+	4+		256

Table 7.20 Grading of agglutination by tube

Grade	Agglutination
Grade 4+	1 big clump
Grade 3+	2 or 3 clumps
Grade 2+	Many small clumps with clear supernatant
Grade 1+	Many small clumps with turbid supernatant granular suspension
Zero clump	Smooth suspension
H	Partial or complete hemolysis (positive reaction)

Add two drops of Rh (D) 5% red cell suspension in all the tubes from 1 to 10.

Incubate all the tubes at 37 °C in water bath for 30 min.

Centrifuge all the ten tubes at 1500 rpm for 1 min.

Examine the tube macroscopically and microscopically for hemagglutination and record the result. The reciprocal of the highest dilution that shows agglutination is the **titer** (Table 7.19).

Prozone phenomenon: In this phenomenon hemagglutination reaction is weaker in the lower dilution and gets stronger in the higher dilution. Example 4 indicates prozone phenomenon in which agglutination is present in higher dilution (256). This is due to the excessive amount of antibody against a small amount of antigen (Table 7.20).

Further Reading

Blood Observational Study Investigators on Behalf of the ANZICS-Clinical Trials Group. Transfusion practice and guidelines in Australian and New Zealand intensive care units. Intensive Care Med. 2010;36:1138–46.

British Committee for Standards in Haematology, Milkins C, Berryman J, Cantwell C, Elliott C, Haggas R, Jones J, Rowley M, Williams M, Win N. Guidelines for pretransfusion compatibility procedures in blood transfusion laboratories. Transfus Med. 2013;23(1):3–5.

Coombs RR, Mourant AE, Race RR. A new test for the detection of weak and "incomplete" Rh agglutinins. Br J Exp Pathol. 1945;26(4):255.

Coombs RR. Historical note: past, present and future of the antiglobulin test. Vox Sanguinis. 1998;74(2):67–73.

Freedman J. False-positive antiglobulin tests in healthy subjects and in hospital patients. J Clin Pathol. 1979;32(10):1014–8.

Gooch A, Parker J, Wray J, Qureshi H. Guideline for blood grouping and antibody testing in pregnancy. Transfus Med. 2007;17(4):252–351.

Judd WJ. Practice guidelines for prenatal and perinatal immunohematology, revisited.

Keir A, Agpalo M, Lieberman L, Callum J. How to use: the direct antiglobulin test in newborns. Arch Dis Childhood Educ Pract. 2015;100(4):198–203.

Parker V, Tormey CA. The direct antiglobulin test: indications, interpretation, and pitfalls. Arch Pathol Lab Med. 2017;141(2):305–10.

Snyder EL, Falast GA. Significance of the direct antiglobulin test. Lab Med. 1985;16(2):89–96.

8 Hemolytic Disease of the Newborn

8.1 Introduction

Hemolytic disease of the newborn (HDN) (also known as erythroblastosis fetalis) is disease that starts in utero and causes jaundice, anemia, and enlargement of the liver and spleen in the mature infant. The degree of severity of the disease ranges from mild to mental retardation, or stillbirth.

- *Hemolytic* means breaking down of red blood cells.
- *Erythroblastosis* refers to making of immature red blood cells.
- *Fetalis* refers to fetus.

HDN caused by Rh(D) incompatibility between the infant and the mother is more common and severe than the ABO incompatibility.

Other fetomaternal incompatibilities that can cause erythroblastosis fetalis involve the Kell, Duffy, Kidd, MNSs, Lutheran, Diego, Xg, P, Ee, and Cc antigen systems, as well as other antigens (including Fy^a and K) which occur in about 0.5% of pregnancies.

During childbirth the Rh-positive red cells of the fetus cross the placenta and enter the maternal blood circulation. However, it may also happen any time, blood cells of the two circulations mix, such as during a miscarriage or abortion, with a fall, or during an invasive prenatal testing procedure (such as an amniocentesis or chorionic villus sampling). If the mother is Rh negative, she is sensitized to produce anti-D. The immune antibody (anti-D) returns to fetal circulation in subsequent pregnancy by crossing the placental barrier. If the red cells of the infant are Rh positive, the immune antibody reacts with the red cells and destroys them. First and second incompatible pregnancies are usually required to sensitize the mother, and consequently the second and subsequent infants are most often affected. The first infant may be affected in case of those women who have received "incompatible" transfusion. Other modes of sensitization are:

Rh-negative mother given Rh-positive blood or blood component.

Rh-negative women who had an abortion with Rh-positive fetus, or suffered from stillbirth with Rh-positive fetus, and any instrumentation in the uterus. Although all pregnant women with incompatible fetus are capable of becoming immunized, 50% of them remain unaffected even when exposed to antigens stimuli.

Pregnant mothers produce IgG red cell antibodies, which can cross the placenta and destroy the baby's red cells, causing hemolytic disease of the newborn (HDN). HDN can occur in first pregnancy, but this is uncommon. Cord blood bilirubin >4 mg/dL indicates severe isoimmunization.

P. S. Ajmani, *Immunohematology and Blood banking*, https://doi.org/10.1007/978-981-15-8435-0_8

HDN can result in severe anemia and neurological damage in absence of treatment.

Clinical presentation of HDN depends upon the severity of red cell lysis. It may develop mild jaundice and anemia to hydrops fetalis (with ascites, pleural and pericardial effusions). Because the placenta clears bilirubin, the chief risk to the fetus is anemia. Extramedullary hematopoiesis (due to anemia) results in hepatosplenomegaly.

In the most severe cases of HDN, the fetus may die in utero or be born with severe anemia that requires replacement of red cells by exchange transfusion.

Anti-Kell (anti-K) antibody produces anemia in the neonate by suppressing marrow erythroid activity, rather than by increased hemolysis of fetal red cells.

There may also be severe neurological damage after birth as a result of a high bilirubin level (kernicterus).

8.1.1 Who Is Affected by Hemolytic Disease of the Newborn?

Babies affected by HDN are usually in a mother's second or higher pregnancy, after she has become sensitized with a first baby.

8.1.2 Pathophysiology of Hemolytic Disease of the Newborn

When the mother's antibodies attack the red blood cells of the fetus, they are broken down and destroyed (hemolysis). This makes the baby anemic. Anemia is dangerous because it limits the ability of the blood to carry oxygen to the baby's organs and tissues, as a result of it:

The baby's body responds to the hemolysis by trying to make more red blood cells very quickly in the bone marrow, liver, and spleen. This causes these organs to get enlarged. The new red blood cells, called erythroblasts, are often immature and are unable to perform the functions of mature red blood cells.

Breakdown of red blood cells results in the formation of bilirubin. Babies are not easily able to get rid of the bilirubin, and it can build up in the blood and other tissues and fluids of the baby's body. This is called hyperbilirubinemia. Because bilirubin has a pigment or coloring, it causes a yellowish tinge of the baby's skin and tissues clinically known as jaundice. The yellow color of the skin depends on the serum bilirubin level. The higher the bilirubin level, the higher the yellow color of the skin.

Signs and symptoms depend upon the severity of the disease process and can range from mild to severe symptoms; however, each baby may experience symptoms differently.

- **During pregnancy**: Mild anemia, hyperbilirubinemia, and jaundice. The placenta helps to eliminate some of the bilirubin, but not all, leading to jaundice.
  - **Severe anemia with enlargement of the liver and spleen**: When these organs and the bone marrow cannot compensate for the fast destruction of red blood cells, severe anemia results, and other organs are affected.
  - **Hydrops fetalis**: This occurs as the baby's organs are unable to handle the anemia. The heart begins to fail, and large amounts of fluid build up in the baby's tissues and organs. A fetus with hydrops is at great risk of being stillborn.
- **After birth**:
  - **Severe hyperbilirubinemia and jaundice**: The baby's liver is unable to cope up the large amount of bilirubin resulting from breakdown of red blood cells, which leads to enlargement of liver and continuation of anemia.
  - **Kernicterus**: It is due to very high level of bilirubin in the brain resulting in seizures, brain damage, deafness, and death.

8.1.2.1 Laboratory Findings

Analysis of the amniotic fluid will reveal yellow discolorization and bilirubin contamination.

Ultrasound of the fetus reveals enlargement of the liver, spleen, or heart and fluid buildup in the fetus's abdomen, around the lungs, or in the scalp.

Box 8.1: Postnatal Presentation

Asphyxia
Pulmonary hypertension
Pallor due to decreased hemoglobin level
Edema (hydrops, due to low serum albumin)
Respiratory distress
Coagulopathies: decreased platelet count and clotting factors
Kernicterus results (from hyperbilirubinemia)
Hypoglycemia (due to hyperinsulinemia from islet cell hyperplasia)

Box 8.2: Fetomaternal Hemorrhage

FMH is less than 0.05 mL in about 50% of cases
FMH is greater than 0.5 mL in about 5% of cases
FMH is greater than 1 mL in about 3% of cases
FMH is >30 mL in up to 0.6% of cases

Box 8.3: Test for Fetomaternal Hemorrhage

Kleihauer–Betke test
Rosette test
Flow cytometry

After birth, symptoms may include the following:

A pale color of the skin may be evident, due to anemia.

Jaundice or yellow coloring of the amniotic fluid, umbilical cord, skin, and eyes may be present. The baby may not look yellow immediately after birth, but jaundice can develop quickly, usually within 24–36 h.

The newborn may have enlarged liver and spleen.

Babies with hydrops fetalis have severe edema (swelling) of the entire body and are extremely pale. They often have difficulty in breathing (Box 8.1).

Risks during labor and delivery include asphyxia and splenic rupture.

8.1.3 Fetomaternal Hemorrhage

Transplacental transfer of fetal erythrocytes into the maternal circulation is one of the complications of pregnancy. When the physiological barrier between the maternal and the fetal circulation is disrupted, the positive pressure gradient may cause fetal erythrocytes to pass into the maternal circulation.

Fetomaternal hemorrhage refers to the entry of fetal blood into the maternal blood stream before or during delivery. FMH occurs normally in minute amounts throughout pregnancy and increases during parturition. It **takes only 0.02–0.05 mL of FMH to isoimmunize the mother.**

The majority of fetal bleeds are less than 5 mL of red blood cells (Box 8.2).

Antibody formation occurs during pregnancy in about 1–1.5% of RhD-negative women carrying RhD-positive infant, despite use of postnatal prophylaxis.

The rate of antibody formation can be reduced to 0.2% or less by the administration of Rh(D) immunoglobulin during pregnancy, at 28 and 34 weeks (antenatal prophylaxis), as well as after delivery (Box 8.3).

Kleihauer–Betke test is highly sensitive, has poor reproducibility, lacks standardization among laboratories, and shows potential sources of error, namely, thickness of the blood films, number of RBCs in a low-power microscope field, number of nonstainable fetal cells, and variations in pH used.

Rosette test: It detects antibody that binds to fetal Rh-positive RBCs forming rosette; the test detects 5 mL Rh-positive fetal RBCs.

Flow cytometry using monoclonal antibodies directed against Hb F has some important advantages over the Kleihauer–Betke test. Flow cytometric methods can accurately distinguish adult F-cells from fetal RBCs; rapidly analyze a greater number of cells, improving quantitative accuracy; are automated, and have greater reproducibility. It detects 0.1% Rh-positive RBCs equivalent to fetomaternal hemorrhage of 15 mL of whole blood.

8.1.4 Acid Elution Test

Principle: Fetal red cells contain Hb F which is resistant to acid elution.

Prepare a thin blood smear from freshly drawn venous or capillary blood of the mother's blood, and allow it to dry for 10 min.

Fix in ethyl alcohol for 5 min.

Rinse the smear with distilled water and allow it to dry.

Prewarm the citric acid–phosphate buffer.

Place 50 mL of the buffer solution into a Coplin jar and cover. Incubate at 37 °C for 5 min.

Smear can be stained either with Leishman stain or hematoxylin and eosin stain or any other stain used in staining blood smear.

Stain the dry smears in acid hematoxylin for 3 min. Rinse with distilled water, and remove as much of the water as possible from the smears by gently tapping one end of the slide on an absorbent material.

Counterstain the smears with erythrosine B for 4 min. Rinse with distilled water, allow to air-dry, and coverslip.

Examine the slides under oil immersion objective.

Hematoxylin will stain white blood cell nuclei and erythrocin will stain the red cells.

The smears are then reviewed microscopically to find the presence of hemoglobin F, and percentage of red blood cells containing fetal hemoglobin may be assessed.

Reticulocytes may resist elution and would, therefore, give the appearance of cells containing hemoglobin F.

The degree of elution of adult hemoglobin may vary from patient to patient.

Normal cells with Hb A will appear as ghost cells, while fetal cells with Hb F will not be affected and retain their hemoglobin and produce pink color.

Ethyl alcohol concentrations above 80% may cause the elution of hemoglobin F, while concentrations below 80% may cause morphologic alterations.

To determine the percentage of red cells containing fetal Hb, the following formula is used:

$$\%\text{of fetal red cells} \times 50 = \text{mL fetomaternal hemorrhage}$$

On the basis of fetomaternal hemorrhage, the physician will decide the amount of anti-D to be administered.

8.2 Laboratory Diagnosis of HDN–Rh

The laboratory diagnosis of HDN can be divided into two: **prenatal** and **postnatal tests.**

8.2.1 Prenatal Test

- **Rh antibody-D titer**: detection of Rh antibody in the mother's blood and its rising titer on repeated intervals
- **Ultrasound**: is indicated to detect enlargement of live, spleen heart or any other organomegaly or fluid buildup in the fetus

It uses high-frequency sound waves and a computer to create images of blood vessels, tissues, and organs. Ultrasound is used to view the functions of internal organs and to assess blood flow through various vessels.

Middle cerebral artery blood flow measurements for pregnancies considered at risk. In case of increasing anti-D titer, middle cerebral artery (MCA) blood flow is measured at intervals of 1–2 weeks depending on the initial blood flow result and patient history, to ascertain high-output heart failure, indicating high risk of anemia. Elevated blood flow for gestational age points out for bilirubin estimation of percutaneous umbilical blood sampling and intrauterine blood transfusion.

8.2.1.1 Amniocentesis

This test is used for bilirubin estimation and to determine chromosomal and genetic defects.

The test involves inserting a needle through the abdominal and uterine wall into the amniotic sac to retrieve a sample of amniotic fluid.

8.2.2 Postnatal Tests

Once a baby is born, diagnostic tests for HDN may include the following:

- ABO grouping
- Rh D grouping
- Rh antibody titer
- Complete blood count
- Serum bilirubin

8.3 Cell-Free Fetal DNA Screening

8.3.1 Specimen Collection for HDN

The specimens used for these tests are clotted blood specimens of the mother (prenatal and postnatal), father (prenatal), and infant (postnatal).

The specimen for testing is obtained from the baby's umbilical cord immediately following birth. A syringe is used to withdraw a specimen to prevent contamination with Wharton's jelly. Wharton's jelly is a gelatinous, water-soluble substance which coats the umbilical cord. The cord blood specimen should be properly labeled with the mother's name, baby identification (by name or family), hospital number, and date.

The cord specimen will be contaminated if the specimen is collected by cutting the cord and allowing the blood to drip in the tube or if the blood is "milked" into the tube. Contamination of blood sample can be removed by 8–10 washings with increased volume (8 mL) of normal saline.

If the cord specimen becomes contaminated with Wharton's jelly, it will cause non-specific agglutination of the cells (false positives). False positive reactions are usually discovered when the ABO and Rh(D) typing is performed. All forward typing tubes are positive, an Rh control is run, and it is also positive, invalidating the test.

8.3.1.1 Prenatal Test

Determine the ABO and Rh group of the mother and father.

If the mother is Rh negative (irrespective of ABO group) and the father is Rh positive, the occurrence of HDN–Rh can be expected.

Test for the presence of anti-D in the mother, especially after second or subsequent pregnancy.

If the test shows immune antibody is present (anti-D), determine the titer, and find out whether there is rising trend of titer. This is done by determining the antibody- D titre, at monthly or two weekly intervals.

8.3.1.2 Postnatal Investigation

ABO and Rh group of the mother and infant.

Direct antiglobulin (Coombs) test of cord blood is strongly positive.

Elution and identification of antibodies are done if the direct Coombs test is positive. This helps in the search for appropriate blood for exchange transfusion.

8.4 Postnatal Diagnosis and Therapy

Indirect serum bilirubin shows rapid rise to very high 30 mg/dL in untreated infants to maximum in 3–5 days.

Increased urine and fecal urobilinogen parallel serum levels.

Direct antiglobulin test positive: The test may become negative within few days of effective exchange transfusion.

Indirect Coombs test on cord blood may be positive because of "free immune" antibody.

At birth little or low anemia but may develop rapidly by third or fourth day. RBC may decrease by 1 million/cu mm/day.

Increased reticulocyte count: 6–40%.

MCV and MCH are increased; MCHC is normal.

Marked increase in nucleated RBCs in peripheral blood (10,000–100,000/cu mm) during first 48 h and decrease within another 48 h.

Polychromatophilia, anisocytosis, and macrocytic RBCs.

In ABO incompatibility marked spherocytosis with increased osmotic fragility.

Thrombocytopenia.

Leucopenia.

Hypoalbuminemia.

Spherocytosis is absent in Rh incompatibility.

Decreased HB F and increased adult Hb.

Late anemia occurs during second to fourth week of life in 5% of those receiving.

8.5 Prevention of Hemolytic Disease of the Newborn by Routine Rh(D) Prophylaxis Guidelines.

HDN can be effectively prevented by administering Rho (D) immunoglobulin (human) for intramuscular (IM) injection. The following criteria must be met:

- **Antenatal**: Routine prophylaxis for all Rh (D)-negative pregnant women (primigravida and multigravida) and weak D (Du)-negative mothers is recommended at 28 weeks and 34 weeks of gestation.
- **Postpartum**: Administer within 72 h of delivery, to Rho (D)- and weak D (Du)-negative mothers who deliver a Rho (D)-positive baby.
- **Administer within 72 h to** Rho (D)-negative, weak D (Du)-negative women who have an ectopic pregnancy, abortion, therapeutic or diagnostic procedure, or trauma with the possibility of fetomaternal hemorrhage.
- If Rh(D) immunoglobulin has not been administered within 72 h, still can be given within 10 days. It may offer some protection.

8.5.1 Dosage of RhIG

Using the estimated volume of fetal bleed determined by the KB test or flow cytometry, the number of vials of RhIG (300 μg) to inject is calculated as follows (Table 8.1):

$$\text{Number of vials of } 300\,\mu g \text{ of RhIG} = \text{Volume of fetal red cells} / 30$$

Prophylactic Rh(D) immunoglobulin may be indicated when RhD-positive platelets are transfused to an Rh(D)-negative recipient, in female children or women of childbearing age.

Dosage of Rh(D) immunoglobulin: For each sensitizing event or at delivery, Rh(D) immunoglobulin 100 IU is sufficient to protect against a fetomaternal hemorrhage (FMH) of 1.0 mL of fetal red cells (2.0 mL whole blood). For example, Rh(D) immunoglobulin 625 IU is sufficient to protect against a FMH of 6 mL of fetal red cells (12 mL of whole blood).

8.6 Treatment for Hemolytic Disease of the Newborn

Specific treatment for hemolytic disease of the newborn depends on:

- Baby's gestational age, overall health, and medical history
- Severity of the disease
- Baby's tolerance for specific medications, procedures, or therapies

Table 8.1 Calculation

Volume of fetal bleed: % fetal cells × maternal blood volume		
Maternal blood volume: 70 mL/kg × weight (kg) (assume 5000 mL if maternal information is unknown)		
Gestation age	**Dose**	**FMT (fetal red cells only)**
<12 weeks	150 mcg	2.5 mL of Rh-positive red cells
>12 weeks	300 mcg	15 mL of Rh-positive red cells

- Expectations for the outcome of the disease process
- Parent's opinion or preference

During pregnancy, treatment for HDN may include:
- Intrauterine blood transfusion of red blood cells into the baby's circulation.
- Early delivery if the fetus develops complications. If the fetus has mature lungs, labor and delivery may be induced to prevent worsening of HDN.

After birth, treatment may include:
- Blood transfusions (for severe anemia)
- Intravenous fluids (for low blood pressure)
- Help for respiratory distress using oxygen, surfactant, or a mechanical breathing machine

Exchange transfusion is indicated to replace the baby's damaged blood with fresh blood. The exchange transfusion helps increase the red blood cell count and lower the levels of bilirubin. An exchange transfusion is done by alternating giving and withdrawing blood in small amounts through a vein or artery. Exchange transfusions may need to be repeated if the bilirubin levels remain high in spite of the previous exchange transfusion.

Intravenous immunoglobulin (IVIG): IVIG is a solution made from blood plasma that contains antibodies to help the baby's immune system. IVIG may help reduce the breakdown of red blood cells and lower bilirubin levels.

Phototherapy of Coombs-positive infant: This procedure decreases the indication of exchange transfusions from 25% to 10%. Phototherapy should be advised after serum bilirubin is more than 10 mg/dL.

8.6.1 Management of HDN

The referral should be made before 20 weeks in those women who have had a history of severely affected baby, unless there is a new partner who is negative for the relevant antigen.

If antibodies are detected, the levels should be monitored frequently throughout the pregnancy in case they increase in titer.

Rising levels are likely to be indicative of HDN developing in the fetus.

Amniocentesis and the level of bilirubin in the amniotic fluid will give a clearer guide to the severity of the disease.

Management of an affected fetus may include intrauterine transfusion, early delivery, phototherapy, and exchange transfusion.

Treatment: Fetal blood transfusions & early indication of delivery the baby.

8.6.2 Hemolytic Disease of the Newborn Caused by ABO Incompatibility

ABO incompatibility causes approximately 2/3 of cases, while Rh incompatibility is less than 1/3 of cases. Rh incompatibility cases are more severe. The association of a type A or B fetus with a type O mother occurs in 15% of pregnancies. However, HDN occurs in only 3% of cases and is severe in only 1%. ABO incompatibility is more often seen in newborns that have type A blood because of the higher frequency of type A compared to type B in most populations. With maternal blood type A and B, isoimmunization does not occur because the naturally occurring antibodies (anti-A and anti-B) are IgM, not IgG. In type O mothers, the antibodies are predominantly IgG, cross the placenta, and can cause hemolysis in the fetus.

If mother and fetus is ABO incompatible, the maternal serum already has the potentially antigenistic blood group antibody; thus the disease more readily occurs in the firstborn infant.

The prerequisites for ABO incompatibility are the (1) mother is O; (2) fetus is of blood group A (more common); and (3) mother carries immune anti-A in circulation (in more than 90% of cases).

The cause of immune anti-A production in the mother with blood group O is not common, and when present, it does not affect the mother. The immune anti-A is, however, capable of crossing the placenta and will react with fetal red cells bearing A antigen. Although HDN–ABO can occur as often as Rh disease, it is frequently so mild as to be missed unless a close clinical check is made.

Hemolysis may develop in fetuses and neonates who are ABO incompatible with their mother. The hemolysis is due to the IgG anti-A or anti-B crossing the placenta and binding to the fetal red cells. Group A babies of group O mothers have a lower mean Hb and a higher mean cord bilirubin than in ABO-compatible pairs. The expression of A and B antigens on neonatal red cells is much weaker than on adult red cells which reduces the number of molecules of IgG which can bind, thus reducing or preventing hemolysis.

8.6.2.1 Clinical Presentation

ABO incompatibility does not present in utero and does not cause hydrops. ABO incompatibility in the newborn generally presents as neonatal jaundice due to a Coombs-positive hemolytic anemia and occurs in 0.5–1% of newborns.

It is estimated that <1% of type O mothers have clinically significant anti-A or anti-B antibody which is IgG. ABO incompatibility with transplacental transfer of IgG anti-A antibody or, more commonly, anti-B antibody has rarely been reported in association with intrauterine hemolysis leading to hydrops fetalis.

ABO incompatibility does not demonstrate any consistent pattern. Thus, the patient's first offspring may have clinically hemolytic disease of the newborn due to ABO incompatibility, while subsequent newborns from the same parents do not have more serious disease.

Rapidly developing anemia is rare: Infant may show jaundice in the first 24 h but rarely requires exchange transfusion for anemia or hyperbilirubinemia. Increasing serial bilirubin level of more than 20 mg/dL is indication of exchange transfusion.

8.6.2.2 Laboratory Findings

Infant's serum shows positive indirect Coombs test.

Infant's RBC shows negative direct Coombs test due to antibody derived from the mother that has crossed placenta.

Direct and indirect Coombs test become normal after fourth day of birth.

Peripheral blood smear will show **marked microspherocytosis**.

Management: To start with the neonate should be given phototherapy and supportive treatment; it should be initiated promptly as jaundice can become severe enough to lead to kernicterus.

Blood units for exchange transfusion should be group O with low-titer anti-A and anti-B.

A two-volume exchange (approximately 170 mL/kg) is most effective in removing bilirubin.

If bilirubin rises again to dangerous levels, a further two-volume exchange should be performed.

8.7 Intrauterine Fetal Blood Transfusion for HDN Disease

An intrauterine transfusion provides blood to an Rh-positive fetus when fetal red blood cells are being destroyed by Rh antibodies followed by Rhc and K or, less commonly, for fetal parvovirus infection is indicated to correct fetal anemia. Intrauterine platelet transfusions are indicated to correct fetal thrombocytopenia caused by platelet alloimmunization.

8.7.1 Principle

A blood transfusion is given to replace fetal red blood cells that are being destroyed by the Rh-sensitized mother's immune system. This treatment is meant to keep the fetus healthy until he or she is mature enough to be delivered.

The aims of intrauterine transfusion (IUT) are to prevent or treat fetal hydrops before the fetus can be delivered and to enable the pregnancy to advance to a gestational age that will ensure survival of the neonate (in practice, up to 36–37 weeks) with as few invasive procedures as possible (because of the risk of fetal loss).

This is achieved by (a) starting the transfusion program as late as safely possible but before hydrops develops and (b) maximizing the intervals between transfusions, by transfusing as large a volume of red cells as is considered safe.

8.7.2 Diagnostic Criteria for Intrauterine Blood Transfusions

Diagnosis of anemia is suggested by Doppler ultrasound of the middle cerebral artery.

Amniocentesis will revealed increased bilirubin level.

Ultrasound shows features of fetal hydrops, such as swollen tissues and organs.

Fetal blood sampling (FBS) shows that the fetus has severe anemia.

8.7.2.1 Procedure

Transfusions can be given through the fetal abdomen or, more commonly, by delivering the blood into the umbilical vein or artery. Umbilical cord vessel transfusion is the preferred method, because it permits better absorption of blood and has a higher survival rate than does transfusion through the abdomen.

An intrauterine fetal blood transfusion is done in the hospital. The mother may have to stay overnight after the procedure.

The mother is sedated, and an ultrasound image is taken to determine the position of the fetus and placenta.

After the mother's abdomen is cleaned with an antiseptic solution, local anesthetic is given injection to numb the abdominal area where the transfusion needle will be inserted.

Medicine may be given to the fetus to temporarily stop fetal movement.

Ultrasound is used to guide the needle through the mother's abdomen into the fetus's abdomen or an umbilical cord vein.

A compatible blood type (usually type O, Rh negative) is delivered into the fetus's umbilical cord blood vessel.

The mother is given antibiotics to prevent infection. She may also be given tocolytic medicine to prevent labor from beginning, though this is unusual.

A short recovery period (approximately 1–3 h) is needed to allow the mother's sedatives to wear off. If the fetus was given medicine to prevent movement, it may be several hours until the mother can feel the fetus moving again.

A sensitized mother's immune system can destroy a large amount of fetal red blood cells, causing severe anemia.

In a severely affected fetus, transfusions are done every 1–4 weeks until the fetus is mature enough to be delivered safely.

8.7.3 Component and Procedure Specification for Red Cell Preparations

Top-up transfusion formula: desired Hb (g/dL) – Actual Hb × weight (kg) × 3 (10–20 mL/kg).

Group O (low-titer hemolysin) or ABO identical with the fetus (if known) and Rh(D) negative.

K-negative blood is recommended to reduce additional maternal alloimmunization risks. In exceptional cases, e.g., for hemolysis because of maternal anti-c, it may be necessary to give RhD-positive, c-negative blood.

IAT crossmatch compatible: with maternal serum and negative for the relevant antigen(s) determined by maternal antibody status.

Less than 5 days old and in citrate phosphate dextrose (CPD) anticoagulant.

Should be CMV seronegative.

Irradiated.

Should have a hematocrit (packed cell volume, PCV) of up to but not more than 0.75.

Cold pRBCs should be warmed to 30 °C and then transfused.

Transfusion amount formula: volume calculated from the formula of **Rodeck and Deans (1999)**:

$$\frac{\text{Desired PCV} - \text{Fetal PCV} \times \text{fetoplacental blood volume}}{\text{Donor PCV} - \text{Desired PCV}}$$

Transfusion rate: 5–10 mL/min.

8.7.4 Platelet Preparations for IUT

In the presence of severe fetal thrombocytopenia, fetal hemorrhage can be prevented by platelet transfusion.

Should be group O Rh(D) negative and test negatively for high-titer anti-A or anti-B (i.e., have a low-titer hemolysin) or group specific and compatible with maternal antibody.

Be human platelet-specific alloantigen (HPA) compatible with maternal antibody; preferably be collected by apheresis. A platelet concentrate derived from whole blood donations is less preferred.

Be irradiated and concentrated to a platelet count of at least 2000 × 10^9/L; be warmed. As the ambient temperature for storing platelet concentrates is 22 °C, there is no need of warming.

Be in a volume calculated from the formula.

Desired platelet increment.

$$\frac{}{\text{Platelet count of concentrate} \times \text{Fetoplacental blood volume}}$$

Be transfused at a rate of 1–5 mL/min (transfused more slowly than red cells because of the increased risk of fetal circulatory stasis and asystole).

Teflon-coated needles should be used because they are considered to allow samples of fetal blood which give more accurate cell count.

The half-life of RBC which is irradiated gets reduced by 4–5 days, and there may be risk of hyperkalemia. Currently there is no recommendation to use the irradiated pRBC in term baby transfusions. In addition, several recent studies found an increased risk for necrotizing enterocolitis (NEC) in neonates after RBC transfusions, the so-called transfusion-associated NEC.

8.7.5 Prognosis After Intrauterine Transfusion Through Umbilical Cord

Fetal survival after transfusion depends upon the severity of the fetus's illness, the method of transfusion, and the professional skill of the treating doctor in that procedure.

More than 90% of fetuses that do not have hydrops survive.

Box 8.4: Risks of Intrauterine Transfusion

Uterine infection
Fetal infection
Preterm labor
Excessive bleeding and mixing of fetal and maternal blood
Leakage of amniotic fluid from the uterus
Fetal death

About 75% of fetuses that have hydrops survive (Box 8.4).

8.8 Neonatal Exchange Transfusion: Indication and Aims

Exchange transfusion may be used to manage severe anemia at birth, particularly in the presence of heart failure, and to treat severe hyperbilirubinemia, caused by HDN.

The aims of an exchange transfusion are:

To lower the bilirubin concentration in the infant's blood to reduce the risk of brain damage (kernicterus).

To remove or dilute out the infants' sensitized red blood cells and circulating maternal antibodies to reduce red cell destruction.

To substitute the infant's non-functional red cells with healthy red cells having adequate oxygen-carrying capacity from a donor.

To Reduce the amount of immune antibodies in the baby blood.

To correct anemia and treat any potential for heart failure while maintaining euvolemia.

Controversial indications such as metabolic disease, septicemia, and disseminated intravascular coagulation (DIC) have not been subjected to adequate clinical evaluation.

Exchange transfusion is a highly specialized procedure associated with a potential for serious adverse events and should be done by well-trained doctor only.

Other indications for exchange transfusion (excluding HDN) disease in front of are:

Table 8.2 In sick premature infants, serum bilirubin >20 mg/dL is the upper limit of normal to indicate exchange transfusion

Birth weight (g)	Serum bilirubin in mg %
<1000	10.00
1001–1250	13.00
1251–1500	15.00
1501–2000	17.00
2001–2500	18.00
>2500	20.00

Box 8.5: Laboratory Criteria for Performing Exchange Transfusion

Criteria	Continue to follow patient	Consider exchange	Perform exchange
Rh antibody titer in mother	<1:64	>1:64	
Cord Hb	>14 g/dL	>12–14 g/dL	<12 g/dL
Cord bilirubin	<4 mg/dL	<4–5 mg/dL	>5 mg/dL
Capillary blood Hb	>12 g/dL	<12 g/dL	<12 g/dL and decreasing in first 24 h
Serum bilirubin	<18 mg/dL	18–20 mg/dL	>34 mg

Cardiopulmonary bypass pumps priming for cardiac surgery and extracorporeal life support (ECLS).

Benefit versus risk: In well babies, the risk of exchange transfusion is usually small, but in preterm babies who are critical, the risks of exchange transfusion are increased, and the procedure must be balanced to the high morbidity associated with bilirubin encephalopathy (Table 8.2 and Box 8.5).

8.8.1 The Compatibility Test in Case of Exchange Transfusion

The newborn infants do not have natural antibodies in their serum; hence ABO group is done by forward grouping only. Compatibility testing of the fetal cells is done with maternal serum.

Table 8.3 ABO group of blood components to be transfused

Patient's ABO group	Choice	Red cells	Platelets	FFP
O	First choice	O	O	O
O	Second choice		A	A
O	Third choice		B	B
O	Fourth choice			AB
A	First choice	A	A	A
A	Second choice	O	B[c] or O[c]	AB
A	Third choice		AB	B[d]
B	First choice	B	B	B
B	Second choice	O	A[b,c] O[c]	AB
B	Third choice		AB	A[d]
AB	First choice	AB	A[c] or B[c]	A[d]
AB	Second choice	A or B	A	A
AB	Third choice	O	O[c]	B[d]

Repeated crossmatching is not necessary prior to transfusion in the first 4 months of life (development of antibodies to red cell antigens is very uncommon in the first 4 months of life).

Use the mother's serum for crossmatch.

Use indirect Coombs test for crossmatch.

Use Rh-negative donor unless both the mother and baby are Rh positive (Table 8.3).

Table 8.4 The choice of blood group for exchange transfusion

Laboratory findings	Blood needed for exchange transfusion
Mother and baby of same blood group	Identical blood group as fetal cells, Rh negative
Blood group of mother and infant is different	Low-titer blood group O
Suitable donor not available	Use incompatible cells with repeated washings
Dire emergency	Use incompatible cells instead of doing nothing

8.8.2 Platelet Transfusion

(a) Group A platelets with the A_2 subgroup do not express significant amounts of A antigen and are therefore preferable to other group A platelets, when transfusing group O and B recipients.
(b) Apheresis platelets that have a **low-titer anti-A/anti-B** pose a lower risk of hemolysis when transfusing ABO-incompatible components.
(c) Plasma components that have **low-titer anti-A/anti-B** pose a lower risk of hemolysis when transfusing ABO-incompatible components (Table 8.4).

Plasma-reduced red cells with a hematocrit of 0.50–0.60 should be suitable for ET for both hyperbilirubinemia and severe anemia. Whole blood, with a hematocrit of 0.35–0.45, and pRBC, with hematocrit of 0.75, are not suitable for exchange transfusion.

Exchanging the estimated volume of the baby's blood in a "single-volume exchange" will remove 75% of red cells, while a double-volume exchange (160–200 mL/kg, depending on gestation) removes 90% of the initial red cells. A double-volume exchange can remove 50% of available intravascular bilirubin.

The pH of a unit of whole blood or plasma-reduced red cells is around 7.0. This does not contribute to acidosis in the infant. Acidosis is more likely to be a result of underlying hypovolemia, sepsis, or hypoxia. "Correction" of pH to physiological levels by the addition of buffer solutions is not indicated .

8.8.3 Component Specifications

Red cells for ET should be group O or ABO compatible with maternal and neonatal plasma,

Rh(D) negative (or Rh-D identical with neonate) O Rh-negative RBCs do not have major blood group antigens so they are not hemolyzed by maternal antibodies that may still be present in the infant's circulation.

Be negative for any red cell antigens to which the mother has antibodies.

Be IAT crossmatch compatible with maternal plasma.

Be <5 days old (to ensure optimal red cell function and low supernatant potassium levels).

Be collected into CPD anticoagulant.

Be CMV seronegative.

Be irradiated and transfused within 24 h of irradiation. Irradiation is essential if the infant has had a previous IUT and is recommended. Irradiation for ET in absence of IUT is not essential if this would lead to clinically significant delay.

Have a hematocrit of 0.50–0.60, to be transfused only after warming at 30 °C. Most clinical units allow the infusate to approximate the ambient temperature while the blood is flowing from the primary pack through the syringes and filters before finally entering the patient's blood circulation.

Volume transfused is usually 80–160 mL/kg for a term infant and 100–200 mL/kg for a preterm infant (i.e., 1–2 × blood volume) depending on the clinical indication.

- **ABO incompatibility**: Use group O, Rh-specific RBCs. These RBCs contain low levels of antibodies and lack antigen that could trigger any circulating maternal antibodies in the newborn. Subsequent transfusions should be done with RBCs that are compatible with that of the mother and infant.
- **Transfusion dose**: 10–20 mL/kg of body weight (Tables 8.5 and 8.6).

Table 8.5 pRBC requirement for very preterm neonate with estimated blood volume of 100 mL/kg

Current Hb	10 mL/kg	15 mL/kg	20 mL/kg
70 g/L	91 g/L	102 g/L	112 g/L
80 g/L	101 g/L	112 g/L	122 g/L
90 g/L	111 g/L	122 g/L	132 g/L

Table 8.6 Term neonate with estimated blood volume of 80 mL/kg

Current Hb	10 mL/kg	15 mL/kg	20 mL/kg
70 g/L	96 g/L	109 g/L	123 g/L
80 g/L	106 g/L	119 g/L	133 g/L
90 g/L	116 g/L	129 g/L	143 g/L

One blood donation is split into five packs of 50 mL each.

In case of HDN–Rh, the use of identical blood group with Rh-negative blood type is used.

For HDN–ABO, incompatibility cases blood group O with Rh-negative is choice.

In either case the donor's blood must be compatible with the mother's serum. If the mother's blood is not available, test the donor's cells with eluate made from the infant's antibody-coated cells. The donor's cells must also be compatible with the infant's serum with the consideration that all the IgG antibodies that came from the mother might not have got attached to red cells.

Stored red blood cells (RBCs) have a predictable packed cell volume of 60% (±2%), so measurement of hematocrit levels is no longer necessary. In order to dilute the RBCs by 10%, fresh frozen plasma (FFP) of suitable type is added. A request for RBCs for exchange transfusions is normally considered an urgent request.

Volume of RBCs and FFP required: The volume required is dependent on the reason for exchange and is determined by the formula below.

Single volume exchange (anemia with normovolemia): Estimated blood volume depends on gestational age and timing of cord clamping ranging from 53 to 105 mL/kg/min. Mean blood volume was 70 mL/kg (early cord clamping) versus 90 mL/kg (delayed cord clamping for infants weighing 480–2060 g. Estimated single blood volume = 85 mL × weight (kg).

Double volume exchange transfusion: This is mainly used for the management of hyperbilirubinemia and hemolytic disease of the newborn, when other methods of treatment such as early and intensive use of phototherapy have been ineffective. Estimated double volume to be exchanged (mL) = estimated blood volume × 2 × infant weight (kg) Preterm/Term infant = 85 mL × 2 × weight (kg) = 170 mL × weight (kg).

Double volume exchange removes about 85% of the infant's red blood cells. At the end of the exchange blood transfusion, the bilirubin should be about 50% of pre-exchange level. It will rebound at about 4 h to 2/3 the pre-exchange level.

When ordering red cells for an exchange transfusion, remember the priming volume of the exchange circuit is approximately 50 mL, so additional RBCs should be ordered.

Procedure for exchange transfusion: Usually a 5 FG umbilical catheter is inserted to a level that allows free flowing withdrawal of the blood.

The preferred method is the isovolumetric or simultaneous exchange where access is via an umbilical venous catheter (blood in) and an umbilical arterial catheter (blood out).

If either umbilical vessel is not available, then the RBCs can be withdrawn via a peripheral arterial cannula and donor RBCs/FFP infused through a venous cannula. Using this method the RBCs are slowly withdrawn from the umbilical arterial catheter (or peripheral arterial line) in pre-determined aliquots with simultaneous replacement of donor RBCs/FFP through the umbilical venous catheter (or **peripheral venous line) using the same** aliquot size.

The process should not be hurried and should take a minimum of 2 h or more depending on the volume of the exchange.

Push–pull method: When using the same catheter, the RBCs and FFP are pushed in and pulled out through the same umbilical venous catheter. The minimum time for this procedure is 2 h or more depending on the volume of the blood to be exchanged.

Rate of exchange: Suggested rate is 30 aliquots over 2 h, that is, 4 min each cycle. This is irrespective of whether the isovolumetric or push–pull method is used. Aliquot volume for double volume exchange: Aliquot volume (mL) = estimated blood volume × 2 × infant weight (kg)/ number of aliquots in 2 h = 85 mL × 2 × weight (kg)/30.

8.8.4 Post-Exchange Transfusion Monitoring

Monitor infant's glucose level during exchange transfusion with heparinized blood and after exchange with citrated blood, as high glucose content of the citrated blood may cause infant hypoglycemia 2 h later.

Monitor infant's blood pH, because pH of donor is low; prefer fresh heparinized blood. In infants Hb of 15 g/dL corresponds to RBC volume of 30 mL/kg body weight. Transfusion of 6 mL of whole blood equals 2 mL of packed RBCs.

Destruction of 1 g of Hb produces 35 mg of bilirubin. Infant with blood volume of 300 mL can have a decrease in Hb of 1 g/dL that may be undetected but may produce 105 mg of bilirubin.

8.8.5 Laboratory Complications of Exchange Transfusion

Electrocytes: Hyperkalemia, hypernatremia, hypocalcemia, acidosis
Clotting: Overheparinization, thrombocytopenia
Infection: Bacteremia, serum hepatitis
Others: Hypoglycemia

8.8.6 Consideration of Other Transfusion Issues

Do not transfuse to replace blood removed for laboratory testing.

Parents must be informed of the need to transfuse.

A volume of 20 mL/kg of packed RBC over 4 hour is recommended.

Consideration may be given to frusemide 1 mg/kg midway through transfusion in infants with critical circulatory status.

Feeds do not need to be suspended routinely during transfusion.

Further Reading

Ahlfors CE, Wennberg RP, Ostrow JD, Tiribelli C. Unbound (free) bilirubin: improving the paradigm for evaluating neonatal jaundice. Clin Chem. 2009;55(7):1288–99.

American Academy of Pediatrics Subcommittee on Hyperbilirubinemia. Management of hyperbilirubinemia in the newborn infant 35 or more weeks of gestation. Pediatrics. 2004;114(1):297. http://pediatrics.aappublications.org/content/114/1/297.full.html.

Arraut A. Erythrocyte alloimmunization and pregnancy: overview, background, pathophysiology. Medscape, 2017-03-09. Archived from https://emedicine.medscape.com/article/273995-overview#:~:text=Overview-,Overview,immunoglobulin%20G%20(IgG)%20antibodies.

Basu S, Kaur R, Kaur G. Hemolytic disease of the fetus and newborn: current trends and perspectives. Asian J Transfus Sci. 2011;5(1):3.

Bell EF, Segar JL. Iowa neonatology handbook, vol. 14, 2009. Retrieved Aug 2006.

Benders MJ, Meinesz JH, Dorrepaal CA, Steendijk P, van Bel F, van de Bor M. Effect of exchange transfusion on brain perfusion and electrocortical brain activity in newborn lambs. Neonatology. 1999;75(2):130–6.

Bhat YR, Pavan Kumar CG. Morbidity of ABO haemolytic disease in the newborn. Paediatr Int Child Health. 2012;32(2):93–6.

Bjerre JV, Petersen JR, Ebbesen F. Surveillance of extreme hyperbilirubinaemia in Denmark. A method to identify the newborn infants. Acta Paediatr. 2008;97(8):1030–4.

Chen HN, Lee ML, Tsao LY. Exchange transfusion using peripheral vessels is safe and effective in newborn infants. Pediatrics. 2008;122(4):e905–10.

Deka D. Intrauterine transfusion. J Fetal Med. 2016;3(1):13–7.

Guidelines RG. Use of anti-D immunoglobulin for Rh prophylaxis. Revised May 2002.

Handbook NN. Jaundice in the first two weeks of life.

Hemolytic Disease of Newborn Treatment at eMedicine. Archived from https://emedicine.medscape.com/article/974349-treatment#:~:text=Apart%20from%20early%20phototherapy%2C%20they,approximately%2025%25%20of%20affected%20neonates.

Jackson JC. Adverse events associated with exchange transfusion in healthy and ill newborns. Pediatrics. 1997;99(5):e7.

Jeon H, Calhoun B, Pothiawala M, Herschel M, Baron BW. Significant ABO hemolytic disease of the newborn in a group B infant with a group A2 mother. Immunohematology. 2000;16(3):105.

Kleihauer E. Demonstration of fetal hemoglobin in erythrocytes of a blood smear. Klin Wochenschr. 1957;35:637–41.

Letsky EA, Leck IN, Bowman SK. Rhesus and other haemolytic diseases. In: Antenatal & neonatal screening, 2000.

Moise KJ Jr. Intrauterine transfusion with red cells and platelets. West J Med. 1993;159(3):318.

Murki S, Kumar P. Blood exchange transfusion for infants with severe neonatal hyperbilirubinemia. In: Seminars in perinatology, vol. 35(3). Philadelphia, PA: W.B. Saunders; 2011. p. 175–84.

Murray NA, Roberts IA. Haemolytic disease of the newborn. Arch Dis Child Fetal Neonatal Ed. 2007;92(2):F83–8.

Pilgrim H, Lloyd-Jones M, Rees A. Routine antenatal anti-D prophylaxis for RhD-negative women: a systematic review and economic evaluation. In: NIHR Health Technology Assessment programme: executive summaries. NIHR Journals Library, 2009.

Ramasethu J, MacDonald MG. Atlas of procedures in neonatology. Philadelphia, PA: Lippincott Williams & Wilkins; 2007.

Robitaille N, Panagopoulos A, Nuyt AM, Hume HA. Exchange transfusion in the infant. In: Handbook of pediatric transfusion medicine, vol. 1. Amsterdam: Academic Press; 2004. p. 159–65.

Shapiro SM. Definition of the clinical spectrum of kernicterus and bilirubin-induced neurologic dysfunction (BIND). J Perinatol. 2005;25(1):54–9.

Team BT, World Health Organization. The clinical use of blood: handbook. Geneva: World Health Organization; 2001.

Thayyil S, Milligan D. Single versus double volume exchange transfusion in jaundiced newborn infants. Cochrane Database Syst Rev. 2006(4).

The Royal Women's Hospital, Melbourne, Exchange transfusion (total & partial): neonatal, 2006. Archived from https://www.rch.org.au/uploadedFiles/Main/Content/neonatal_rch/EXCHANGE_TRANSFUSION.pdf.

Urbaniak SJ, Greiss MA. RhD haemolytic disease of the fetus and the newborn. Blood Rev. 2000;14(1):44–61.

Usha KK, Sulochana PV. Detection of high risk pregnancies with relation to ABO haemolytic disease of newborn. Indian J Pediatr. 1998;65(6):863–5.

White J, Qureshi H, Massey E, Needs M, Byrne G, Daniels G, Allard S. British Committee for Standards in Haematology. Guideline for blood grouping and red cell antibody testing in pregnancy. Transfus Med. 2016;26(4):246–63.

9 History of Blood Transfusion

9.1 The Beginning

People have always been fascinated by blood. Ancient Egyptians bathed in it, aristocrats drank it, authors and playwrights used it as themes, and modern humanity transfuses it. The road to an efficient, safe, and uncomplicated transfusion technique has been rather difficult, but great progress has been made.

In 400 BC Hippocrates, a Greek physician, postulated that the body is comprised of four humors—blood, phlegm, black bile, and yellow bile—and their imbalance causes disease.

In 350 BC Aristotle, a Greek philosopher, believed that the heart is the central organ of the body. Following dissections of many different animals, Aristotle presumes the heart is a three-chambered organ, even in humans.

In 350 BC Galen (Claudius Galenus), a Greek physician, described the anatomy of the human body and includes a reference to "bright" and "dark" blood from separate "channels in the body" which interconnect. Galen also mentions the "liver" as the origin of blood and the kidneys as a filter. Although incorrect in many details, his descriptions formed the basis for all blood circulation studies for centuries.

In 1492, blood was taken from three young men and given to the stricken Pope Innocent VII in the hope of curing him. Unfortunately, all four died. Although the outcome of this event was unsatisfactory, it is the first time a blood transfusion was recorded.

The first research into blood transfusion dates back to the seventeenth century when British physician William Harvey fully described the circulation and properties of blood in his *De Motu Cordis* in 1628. The first blood transfusions were also attempted around this time, although these were unsuccessful and proved fatal in humans.

After being banned for more than 150 years, the use of blood transfusion was revived during the late eighteenth century.

In 1658 microscopist Jan Swammerdam observed and described the red blood cells.

9.2 The First Transfusions

- 1665 The first successful blood transfusion recorded was performed by British physician Richard Lower in 1665, when he bled a dog almost to death and then revived the animal by transfusing blood from another dog via a tied artery.
- 1667 Jean-Baptiste Denis in France and Richard Lower and Edmund King in England separately reported successful transfusions from sheep to human.
- In 1818 the first successful man to man blood transfusion was performed by British obstetri-

P. S. Ajmani, *Immunohematology and Blood banking*, https://doi.org/10.1007/978-981-15-8435-0_9

cian James Blundell. He successfully transfused human blood to a patient who had hemorrhage during childbirth.
- 1873–1880 US physicians attempted transfusing milk from cows, goats, and humans.
- 1884 Saline infusion replaced milk as a "blood substitute" due to the increased frequency of adverse reactions to milk.

9.3 Dawn of a New Era

- 1901 Karl Landsteiner, an Austrian physician, discovered the three main human blood groups A, B, and C. (He later changes C to O.)
- 1902 A fourth main blood type, AB, was found by A. Decastrello and A. Sturli.
- 1907 Ludvig Hektoen suggested that the safety of transfusion might be improved by crossmatching blood between donors and patients to exclude incompatible mixtures.
- 1907 Reuben Ottenberg performed the first blood transfusion using blood typing and crossmatching.
- 1908 Alexis Carrel, a French surgeon, devised a way to prevent blood clotting. His method involved surgically joining an artery in the donor directly to a vein in the recipient. This procedure, not feasible for blood transfusion, paved the way for successful organ transplantation, for which Carrel received the Nobel Prize in 1912.
- 1912 Roger Lee, an American physician, and P. White formulated and developed the "Lee–White" clotting time. Lee further demonstrated that blood from all groups can be given to group AB patients.
- 1914 Long-term anticoagulants, among them sodium citrate, were developed, allowing longer preservation of blood.
- 1915 Luis Agate, an Argentinean physician; Albert Hustin, Belgian physician; and Richard Lewiston, New York physician, independently described methods for using anticoagulated blood.
- 1915 Francis Rous and J. R. Turner introduced the Rous–Turner solution: a citrate–glucose solution that permitted storage of blood for several days after collection.
- 1920 John and Dr. Charles drew revolutionized storage and distribution of blood.
- 1922 Percy Lane Oliver started the first blood donor service. He recruits volunteers who agree to be on 24-h call and to travel to local hospitals to give blood as the need arises.
- 1926 The British Red Cross instituted the first human blood transfusion service in the world.
- 1935 A group of anesthesiologists at the Mayo Clinic in Rochester, MN, were the first to begin storing preserved blood and utilizing it for transfusions.
- 1935 W. B. Murphy first used plastic bag to store blood.
- 1937 Dr. Bernard Fantus coined the term "blood bank" to describe a facility for blood donation, collection, and preservation.
- 1939 India's first blood bank was established in a school of tropical medicine, Kolkata, by Dr. Upendranath Brahmachari chairman of Bengal Red Cross Society.
- 1939 Coombs, Mourant, and Race described the use of anti-human globulin to identify incomplete antibodies. The process became known as the Coombs test, also known as the antiglobulin test.
- 1939 Levine and Stetson defined D antigen (Rh factor).
- 1940 Landsteiner and Weiner discovered anti-Rh (named after Rhesus monkey) agglutinated 85%
- 1940 The US government established a national blood collection program.

9.4 The Blood Bank

- 1940 Edwin Cohn developed cold ethanol fractionation, the process of breaking down plasma into components and products. Albumin, gamma globulin, and fibrinogen are isolated and become available for clinical use.
- 1940 John Elliott developed the first blood container, a vacuum bottle extensively used by the Red Cross.

- 1940 Early blood processing program for relief of English war victims, called Plasma for Britain, began under the direction of Charles R. Drew, MD.
- 1940 Freeze-dried plasma was developed.
- 1940 Charles Drew started the "Blood for Britain" program leading to the manufacture of large quantities of dried plasma.
- 1941 The American Red Cross agreed to organize a civilian blood donor service to collect blood plasma for the war effort.
- 1944 Dried plasma became a vital element in the treatment of wounded soldiers during the world war. The Red Cross ended its World War II blood program for the military after collecting more than 13 million pints.
- 1946 The Kell blood group was discovered. It is named for a Mrs. Kelleher, whose child had hemolytic disease of the newborn because of a maternal/fetal blood type mismatch.
- 1947 Syphilis testing is performed on each unit of blood.
- 1948 The Red Cross began the first nationwide blood program for civilians by opening its first collection center in Rochester, NY.
- 1949 The US blood system is comprised of 1500 hospital blood banks, 46 community blood centers, and 31 American Red Cross regional blood centers.
- 1950 Carl Walter and W. P. Murphy introduced the plastic bag for blood collection.
- 1950 Audrey Smith reports the use of glycerol cryoprotectant for red blood cells.
- 1950 The USA enters Korean War. Red Cross became blood collection agency for military during Korean War.
- 1950 The Duffy blood group was discovered. It is named for a patient with hemophilia who received multiple blood transfusions and was the first known producer of anti-Duffy antibodies.
- 1951 The Kidd blood group was discovered. It is named after a Mrs. Kidd, who was found to have produced antibodies targeted against a red blood cell antigen during her pregnancy, causing hemolytic disease of the newborn in her child.
- 1953 Development of the refrigerated centrifuge began to further expedite blood component therapy.
- 1954 The blood product cryoprecipitate was developed for people suffering from hemophilia.
- 1955 The Diego blood group was discovered. It is named for a Mrs. Diego, whose child had hemolytic disease of the newborn because of a maternal/fetal blood type mismatch.
- 1956 Establishment of national blood clearing house
- 1956 Products made from blood plasma were developed to treat diseases such as chicken pox.
- 1957 The American Association of Blood Banks for its committee on inspection and accreditation to monitor the implementation of standards for blood banking
- 1957 Platelet concentrates are recognized for reducing the mortality from hemorrhage in cancer patients.
- 1960 A. Solomon and J. L. Fahey reported the first therapeutic plasmapheresis procedure.
- 1964 Plasmapheresis is introduced as a means of collecting plasma for fractionation.
- In 1964, infection of jaundice through blood transfusion was confirmed.
- 1967 American National Red Cross Board of Governors received report that national headquarters will host a national Rare Blood Donor Registry for blood types occurring less than once in 200 people.
- 1969 S. Murphy and F. Gardner demonstrated the feasibility of storing platelets at room temperature, revolutionizing platelet transfusion therapy.
- 1970 US blood banks move toward an all-volunteer blood donor system.
- 1971 Hepatitis B surface antigen (HbsAg) testing of donated blood began.
- 1972 The Red Cross calls for national blood policy, which the federal government sets up in 1974, supporting standardized practices and an end to paid donations.

- 1972 Apheresis is used to extract one cellular component, returning the rest of the blood to the donor.
- 1972 The Food and Drug Administration (FDA) began to regulate all 7000 US blood and plasma centers.
- 1972 Apheresis was used to extract one cellular component.
- 1978 FDA requires blood bags to be labeled "paid" or "volunteer."
- 1979 A new anticoagulant preservative, CPDA-1, which extends the shelf life of whole blood and red blood cells to 35 days was introduced. Additive solutions extend shelf life of red blood cells to 42 days.
- 1979 Red Cross Blood Services regions began testing all newly donated blood.
- 1987 The Red Cross opens its Holland Laboratory dedicated to biomedical research.
- 1990 Hepatitis C testing was introduced.
- 1992 Testing of donor blood for HIV 1 and HIV 2 antibodies (anti-HIV 1 and anti-HIV 2) was implemented.
- 1992 First National Testing Laboratory, applying standardized tests to ensure safety of Red Cross blood products, opened in Dedham, Mass. Today, the Red Cross performed a dozen tests on each of more than six million blood donations a year in five state-of-the-art standardized national testing laboratories (NTLs).
- 1993 First edition of the *Guidelines for the Blood Transfusion Services in the United Kingdom*, also known as the *Red Book*, was published.
- 1994 The European Association of the Plasma Products Industry, a trade group representing blood manufacturers in Europe and the UK, was founded.
- 1996 Variant Creutzfeldt–Jakob disease (vCJD) was identified. The clinical, epidemiological, neuropathological, and experimental data all point to variant CJD being caused by the same strain of prion as bovine spongiform encephalopathy (BSE). This is a different strain of prion from those seen in sporadic CJD.
- 1998 The Supreme Court of India passed judgment on blood transfusion and blood banking in India. The Supreme Court banned buying blood from commercial sellers in India. The National Blood Transfusion Council and State Blood Transfusion Councils were established for improvement of blood banking services in the country.
- 1998 The UK Department of Health (DH) publishes its circular *Better Blood Transfusion*. The circular recommendations make evidence-based practice for blood transfusion mandatory for all NHS hospitals and in particular recommend the introduction of perioperative cell salvage (PCS).
- 1999 Leucodepletion was applied to all blood and component donations in the UK.
- 2002 Nucleic acid amplification test (NAT) for HIV and hepatitis C virus (HCV) was licensed by the Food and Drug Administration.
- 2003 First-ever National Blood Foundation forum united leaders in blood banking and transfusion medicine.
- 2003 FDA issued final guidance regarding "Revised Recommendations for the Assessment of Donor Suitability and Blood and Blood Product Safety in Cases of Known or Suspected West Nile Virus Infection."
- 2003 First West Nile Virus-positive unit of blood intercepted.
- 2003 Guidance on Implementation of New Bacteria Reduction and Detection Standard was issued.
- 2004 AABB received $2.4 Million CDC grant to reduce transfusion-transmitted HIV in Africa and South America.
- 2005 FDA cleared apheresis platelets collected with certain systems for routine storage and patient transfusion up to 7 days when tested with a microbial detection system release test.
- 2005 FDA's Center for Biologics Evaluation and Research published compliance program guidance for inspection of human cells, tissues, and cellular and tissue-based products (HCT/Ps).
- 2005 FDA approved the first West Nile virus (WNV) blood test to screen donors of blood, organs, cells, and tissues.

Further Reading

Durand JK, Willis MS. Karl Landsteiner, MD: transfusion medicine. Lab Med. 2010;41(1):53–5.

Elizabeth Y. First blood transfusion: a history. Journal Storage: Digital Library (JSTOR: Daily), 2015.

Giangrande PL. The history of blood transfusion. Br J Haematol. 2000;110(4):758–67.

Sri Kantha S. The blood revolution initiated by the famous footnote of Karl Landsteiner's 1900 paper.

Starr D. Blood: an epic history of medicine and commerce. New York: Knopf; 2012.

10 Massive Blood Transfusion

10.1 Massive Blood Transfusion (MBT)

Hemorrhage is the most common cause of potentially preventable deaths in trauma and non-trauma patients. Rapid transfusion of large volumes of blood products is required in situations like battle field injury, road side accidents, polytrauma, major surgeries, gastrointestinal hemorrhage, rupture of gastric ulcer, obstetric hemorrhage, ectopic pregnancy, placenta previa, placental abruption, and rupture of aneurysm, with development of hemorrhagic shock which may lead to a unique set of complications. Massive transfusion protocols (MTPs) have been designed for timely recognition and efficient management to accelerate the release of blood products for successful outcomes after major blood loss but can result in waste if activated inappropriately.

Injuries are serious problems common to all in modern-day societies. Exsanguinating hemorrhage is the most common cause of mortality in the first hour of arrival to a trauma center and accounts for almost 50% of deaths in the first 24 h of these patients; 25–40% will be coagulopathic at the time of admission to the trauma center. This coagulopathy can result an increase in mortality rate, and early correction of this coagulopathy could reduce blood product usage and mortality. It consumes 70% of the total blood transfused to trauma patients.

Massive blood transfusion best clinically defined as:

- Continuing blood loss of 150 mL/min for first 30 min
- Continuing blood loss of 1.5 mL/kg/min over 30 min
- Pediatric patient requiring >15 mL/kg of PRBCs in first hour of resuscitation

Historical definition of massive blood transfusion:

- Loss of entire blood volume equivalent within 24 h
- Loss of 50% of blood volume within 3 h
- The administration of ≥10 units of packed red blood cells (pRBC) to a patient in first 12 h
- Administration of more than 4 pRBC concentrates within 1 h
- Any transfusion which involves the administration of blood in which 10% of the blood volume is replaced in 10 min or less (50 mL/min in adult and 15 mL in neonates)

Historical definition is of little importance in clinical practice because trauma patients bleed to death more quickly than initiation of treatment

P. S. Ajmani, *Immunohematology and Blood banking*, https://doi.org/10.1007/978-981-15-8435-0_10

and secondly the resultant shock causes a coagulopathy and ultimately reduces the survival rate.

Normal blood volume being approximately 7% of ideal body weight in adults and 8–9% in children.

10.1.1 Pathophysiology

The body responds to acute blood loss with four basic compensatory mechanisms. Knowledge of these mechanisms allows physicians to adequately assess for the need for blood transfusion.

1. The first response is increased cardiac output. Stroke volume increases due to decreased systemic vascular resistance (SVR). Due to the diminished viscosity of the blood SVR decreases.
2. Increase in cardiac output results in increased blood supply to vital organs, or organs that have higher oxygen extraction ratios. **This (blood flow redistribution) is the primary mechanism for cardiac compensation to anemia**. This is aided by an increase in oxygen extraction from hemoglobin. The heart itself has limited ability to increase its oxygen extraction, but compensates due to its increased coronary blood flow.
3. The oxygen-hemoglobin dissociation curve adjusts during periods of anemia. Anemia causes an increase in 2,3-DPG, which shifts this curve to the right. This decreases the affinity of hemoglobin for oxygen, which facilitates oxygen extraction by tissues.
4. During acute surgical blood loss, the adrenergic nervous system is stimulated, which leads to vasoconstriction and tachycardia.

10.1.2 Definition of Massive Blood Transfusion in Children's

In older, adult-sized children, defined as greater than 10 units of pRBCs in 24 h.

In smaller children's:

1. Packed red blood cell (pRBC) transfusion of 50% of total blood volume (TBV) in 3 h
2. Packed RBC transfusion of 100% total blood volume in 3 h
3. Packed RBC transfusion of >10% of total blood volume per minute

Total blood volume in children's:

Generally accepted blood volume conversion factors are:

- Premature neonate 100 mL/kg for
- Mature neonates 90 mL/kg
- Infants and 80 mL/kg
- Older children 70–80 mL/kg

Massive blood loss in the pediatric patient, often from blunt trauma, can be difficult to assess.

The parameters of assessing pediatric massive blood loss are similar to adults.

However, pediatric patients have good physiological reserve, maintaining arterial pressure even after a loss of 25–40% of blood volume.

Massive obstetric hemorrhage defined as blood loss that is "uncontrolled" and "ongoing" with a rate of blood loss of 150 mL/min or more per minute within 30 min (Box 10.1).

10.1.3 Postpartum Hemorrhage (PPH)

Postpartum hemorrhage (PPH) is defined as blood loss of greater than 500 mL after giving birth vaginally or a blood loss of more than 1000 mL after cesarean section within the first 24 h following childbirth. Hemorrhage most commonly occurs after the placenta is delivered, but it can occur later as well.

Minor Primary Postpartum Hemorrhage: The loss of 500–1000 mL of blood from the genital tract within 24 h of the birth of a baby.

Major Primary Postpartum Hemorrhage: The loss of over 1000 mL of blood from the

Box 10.1: Types of Obstetric Hemorrhage

Primary postpartum hemorrhage
Secondary PPH
Massive obstetric hemorrhage

genital tract within 24 h of the birth of a baby. The loss of more than 500 mL with clinical shock is also major primary postpartum hemorrhage.

Secondary PPH is defined as abnormal or excessive bleeding from the birth canal between 24 h and 6 weeks postnatally. Secondary PPH can be minor 500–1000 mL or major >1000 mL. It is often due to erosion of a vessel from a spreading infection and is most often seen when a heavily contaminated wound is closed primarily.

Definition of PPH assumes clinical significance in light of "readiness for resuscitation" in response to blood loss 500–1000 mL, but "a full protocol of measures" when the blood loss reaches 1000 mL, or there are clinical signs of shock.

At term blood flow to the uterus is around 700 mL/min and bleeding can be dramatic and rapidly fatal. Risk factors for obstetric hemorrhage include placenta previa, placental abruption, and postpartum hemorrhage (most commonly due to uterine atony).

A healthy woman has a 30–50% increase in blood volume in a normal single on pregnancy and is much more tolerant of blood loss than a woman who has pre-existing anemia, an underlying cardiac condition, or a condition secondary to dehydration or preeclampsia.

Women with a low body mass index also have a lower blood volume, tend to have fewer reserves to withstand significant blood loss, and so are likely to experience adverse physiological effects sooner.

Every obstetric unit should have a current protocol for major obstetric hemorrhage, and all staff should be trained to follow it.

10.1.3.1 Pathophysiology of Postpartum Hemorrhage

Once a baby is delivered, the uterus normally continues to contract (tightening of uterine muscles) and expels the placenta. After the placenta is delivered, these contractions help compress the bleeding vessels in the area where the placenta was attached. If the uterus does not contract strongly enough, called uterine atony, these blood vessels bleed freely and hemorrhage occurs. This is the most common cause of postpartum hemorrhage. If small pieces of the placenta remain attached, bleeding is also likely.

Estimation of blood loss during postpartum hemorrhage (PPH): It can be done by counting the number of saturated pads or by weighing of packs and sponges used to absorb blood; 1 mL of blood weighs approximately (1 g), but this method has been underestimated with a 30–50% of blood loss, especially for larger volumes.

10.2 Massive Blood Transfusion in Battle Field Injury (Trauma Induced)

Massive transfusion is generally necessary in severely injured military personnel, CRP forces, border security forces, or patients with multiple injuries. Such patients often require multiple, complex surgical procedures. A rational blood transfusion protocol can improve the outcome of surgery, whereas unreasonably excessive transfusion can lead to mortality, predominantly due to DIC, acidosis, and hypothermia.

Rapid loss of blood leading to **decompensation** and **circulatory failure** despite volume replacement and interventional treatment (Tables 10.1, 10.2 and Box 10.2).

Table 10.1 Clinical signs and symptoms of volume of blood loss

% Blood loss	Systolic BP	Signs and symptoms
10–15%	Normal	Postural hypotension
15–30%	Slight fall	Pulse rate, thirst weakness
30–40%	60–80	Pallor, oliguria, confusion
40+%	40–60	Anuria, air hunger, coma, and death

Table 10.2 Signs and symptoms of inadequate oxygen delivery

$ScO_2 < 70\%$ ($N = 80\%$) (central line)	Mental status alteration
$SvO_2 < 65\%$ (Nl = 75%) (pa catheter)	Dyspnea
Low cerebral or tissue oximetry	Chest pain
Base deficit	New arrhythmias
Lactic acidosis	Tachycardia (not from hypovolemia)
ECG: ST elevation in anterior lead	Decreased LV contractility

Box 10.2: Methods for Volume Status Assessment in Trauma, Predictor of Massive Bleeding

Assessment of blood consumption (ABC) score
Clinical criteria at the time of admission
Clinical criteria for trauma or non-trauma patient's
Laboratory criteria

Table 10.3 Assessment of blood consumption (ABC) score

Parameters	Yes	No	Point
Penetrating injury	1	0	1
Arrival systolic BP < 90	1	0	1
Arrival heart rate > 120	1	0	1
Positive FAST	1	0	1

Table 10.4 Criteria (1 point assigned for each item) interpretation

Score	Need of transfusion
0–1	Massive transfusion unlikely
3	Massive transfusion likely
4	Massive transfusion needed
2	"Positive" to predict MT

Assessment of blood consumption (ABC) score: The ABC score is a valid instrument to predict MT early in the patient's care and across various demographically diverse trauma centers. It has become a widely accepted score for MTP activation at three levels:

ABC score determines need for massive transfusion in trauma patients based on non-laboratory and non-weighted parameters. Early initiation of massive transfusion has been shown to improve survival in critical trauma patients. The ABC score reduces delay in determining need for massive transfusion in a trauma patient while also providing consistency in appropriateness of transfusion by reducing practice variations among providers. The score is calculated by assigning a value (0 or 1) to each of the four parameters (Tables 10.3 and 10.4).

Sensitivity and specificity for the ABC score predicting MT ranged from 70% to 85% and from 65% to 86%, respectively. The score can be repeated as the patient's clinical condition changes very fast.

10.2.1 Focused Assessment with Sonography for Trauma (FAST)

In trauma medicine, there is often a need for quick, qualitative assessment of a patient. The Focused Assessment with Sonography in Trauma (FAST) and extended Focused Assessment with Sonography for Trauma (eFAST) exams are the current standard for rapid evaluation of trauma patients. Training for carrying out eFAST assessment requires practitioners to understand the 3D structures of the body Thais seen in the 2D ultrasound image.

Indications for the eFAST exams include:

- Abdominal and thoracic injuries due to blunt and penetrating trauma.
- Undifferentiated shock and hypotension (as part of the rapid ultrasound for shock and hypotension (RUSH)).
- Decision to operate cannot depend alone on the FAST result, and negative FAST does not exclude injury. This parameter is meant to help with interpretation of FAST findings, which are at least partially dependent on the radiologist skills and sonographic technique.

Rapid ultrasound in shock (RUSH): it was first introduced in 2006 by Weingart SD and is a recently reported emergency ultrasound protocol designed to help clinicians better recognize distinctive shock etiologies in a short time. Patients with hypotension or shock have high mortality rates, and traditional physical exam techniques can be misleading. The mnemonic of the RUSH protocol—pump, tank, and pipes—was created as a physiological roadmap for clinicians to easily remember in the heat of resuscitation. It involves a three-part bedside physiologic assessment simplified as "the pump," "the tank," and "the pipes." The first step in evaluation of the patient in shock is determination of cardiac status, termed for simplicity "the pump." The second part of the RUSH protocol focuses on the determination of the effective intravascular volume status, which will be referred to as "the tank." The pipes is the third and final step in the RUSH exam is to examine "the pipes," looking first at the arterial side of the circulatory system, and, secondly, at the venous side. Ultrasound is ideal for the evaluation of critically ill patients in shock, and ACEP guidelines now delineate a new category of ultrasound (US) "resuscitative." Bedside ultrasound (US) allows for direct visualization of pathology and differentiation of shock states (Box 10.3).

Adult patients with likelihood of requiring transfusion of >10 units of pRBCs within the first 12 h of resuscitation or pediatric patient with the likelihood of requiring transfusion of >0.1 units/kg of pRBCs within the first 12 h of resuscitation.

Clinical criteria for trauma or nonsurgical hemorrhage: Continued blood loss of 150 mL/min for 30 min (Box 10.4).

pH: Healthy human arterial blood pH varies between 7.35 and 7.45. Low pH of blood is due to increased production of hydrogen ions by the body or the inability of the body to form bicarbonate (HCO_3^-) in the kidney. Acidosis refers to a process that causes a low pH in blood and tissues.

Box 10.3: Clinical Criteria for Massive Transfusion Protocol at the Time of Admission

Systole blood pressure <70 mmHg
Temperature <34 °C
Estimated blood loss >1000 mL
The Injury Severity Score (ISS) is >25
Systole <90 mmHg despite of infusion of >3 L of crystalloid 50 mL/kg
Heart rate >120/min

Box 10.4: Laboratory Criteria for Massive Transfusion Protocol

Base deficit >8
INR >1.4
Prothrombin time (PT) >18 s
Partial prothrombin time (PTT) >60 s
Admission Hct value <30
pH 7.1

In trauma patients, the admission value of arterial base deficit stratifies severity of injuries, predicts complications, and is correlated with arterial lactate concentration. In theory, elevated base deficit and lactate concentrations after shock are related to oxygen transport imbalance at the cellular level. A negative number is called a base deficit and indicates a metabolic acidosis.

The most severe injuries occur less frequently.

The Abbreviated Injury Scale (AIS) is an anatomical scoring system that provides an overall score for patients with multiple injuries. It has the advantage of having a direct link to ICD 9 CM classifications of injury (Tables 10.5 and 10.6).

Each injury is assigned an AIS score on an ordinal scale ranging from 1 (minor injury) to 6 (maximum injury, possibly lethal). In multiple injured patients, the highest AIS are known as the maximum AIS (MAIS). If an injury is assigned an AIS of 6 (unsurvivable injury), the AIS score

Table 10.5 AIS: Body region

AIS code	Body region
1	Head
2	Face
3	Neck
4	Thorax
5	Abdomen
6	Spine
7	Upper extremity
8	Lower extremity
9	Unspecified

Table 10.6 AIS Severity Component

Injury severity description	Score	Example
Minor	1	Superficial laceration
Moderate	2	Fracture sternum
Serious, not life-threatening	3	Open fracture humerus
Severe, life-threatening	4	Tracheal perforation
Critical, survival uncertain	5	Rupture spleen
Maximum, actually untreatable	6	Severance of aorta

Box 10.5: Implicitly Based on Four Criteria

Threat to life
Permanent impairment
Treatment period
Energy dissipation

is automatically assigned to 75. The AIS score is virtually the only anatomical scoring system in use and correlates linearly with mortality, morbidity, hospital stay, and other measures of severity. A major trauma (or multiple traumas) is defined as the Injury Severity Score being greater than 15. Score of 16–24 indicates two serious or one severe injury (Box 10.5).

Acute coagulopathy of trauma due to:

- Massive tissue damage.
- Hypoxia.
- Acidosis.
- Hypothermia.
- Dilution.
- Thrombomodulin generated in shock inhibits fibrinogen formation and disinhibits fibrinolysis.
- Presence of two or more factors: 75% sensitive and 86% specific to predict need of MT.

Different causes of coagulopathy in massive blood loss:

- Trauma induced.
- Coagulopathy due to cardio pulmonary bypass (CPB).
- Coagulopathy due to postpartum hemorrhage.

10.2.2 Pathophysiology of Trauma-Induced Coagulopathy

Trauma due to any cause is a leading cause of death, with uncontrolled bleeding and exsanguination being the primary causes of preventable deaths during the first 24 h following trauma. Death usually occurs within the first 6 h after injury. Twenty-five percent of patients after trauma are already in hemodynamic and hemostatic depletion. This early manifestation of hemostatic depletion is referred to as the coagulopathy of trauma, which may distinguish as (1) acute traumatic coagulopathy (ATC) and (2) iatrogenic coagulopathy (IC).

The principle drivers of acute traumatic coagulopathy (ATC) have been characterized by tissue trauma, inflammation, hypoperfusion, shock, and the acute activation of the neurohumoral system. Hypoperfusion leads to an activation of protein C with cleavage of activated factors V and VIII and the inhibition of plasminogen activator inhibitor-1 (PAI-1), with subsequent fibrinolysis. Endothelial damage and activation results in Weibel–Palade body degradation and glycocalyx shedding associated with autoheparinization.

In contrast, (IC) iatrogenic coagulopathy occurs secondary to uncritical volume therapy, leading to acidosis, hypothermia, and hemodilution. This coagulopathy may, then, be an integral part of the "vicious cycle" when combined with acidosis and hypothermia. The awareness of the specific pathophysiology and of the principle drivers underlying the coagulopathy of trauma by the treating physician is paramount. It has been shown that early recognition prompted by appropriate and aggressive management can correct coagulopathy, control bleeding, reduce blood product use, and improve outcome.

The lethal triad of acidosis, hypothermia, and coagulopathy associated with MT is associated with a high mortality rate. Blood transfusion in trauma surgery and critical care has been identified as an independent predictor of multiple organ failure, systemic inflammatory response syndrome, increased infection, and increased mortality in multiple studies. Once definitive control of hemorrhage has been established, a restrictive approach to blood transfusion should be implemented to minimize further complications.

Hypovolemic shock due to massive hemorrhage is a common clinical scenario resulting in tissue ischemia and acidosis. Hyperkalemia, therefore, may be present in patients with hypovolemia, acidosis, and major tissue trauma even without massive transfusion (Box 10.6).

Box 10.6: Risk Factors Likelihood of Coagulopathy in Patients with Shock

45% if INR is above 1.5
25% if platelets count is <150,000/cu mm
30% if fibrinogen <1.0

Massive transfusion risk identified by:

- Prehospital shock index (SI): SI = Heart rate/systole BP.
- Normal shock index = <0.7.

Coagulopathy due to cardiopulmonary bypass (CPB): Heparin is given in high doses before CPB and hypothermia lead to platelet dysfunction that has been shown to be a major cause for bleeding in patients on CPB. It is further exaggerated by extensive surgical trauma, prolonged blood contact with the CPB circuit.

Coagulopathy due to postpartum hemorrhage: fibrinogen deficiency is the major cause of coagulation abnormality associated with obstetric bleeding which may be compounded by dilutional coagulopathy and hyperfibrinolysis.

10.2.3 Laboratory Test for Uncontrollable Hemorrhage

Prothrombin time: normal value 10–14 s. Higher value indicates uncontrolled bleeding.

PTT: Normal value 30–40 s.

aPTT: more than 70 s (signifies spontaneous bleeding).

10.3 Problems Due to Massive Blood Transfusion

Citrate intoxication is a common complication after massive blood transfusions and often presents itself as metabolic alkalosis. Citrate, which is present as an anticoagulant in blood bags (approximately 3 g), metabolized to bicarbonate, and this conversion happens predominantly in the liver. It is therefore unnecessary to attempt to neutralize the acid load of transfusion. A healthy adult can metabolize this load in 5 min. However, hypoperfusion or hypothermia associated with massive blood loss can decrease this rate of metabolism leading to citrate toxicity. There is very little citrate in red cell concentrates.

Management of citrate intoxication:

- If there is prolongation of PT, give ABO compatible fresh frozen plasma in a dose of 15 mL/kg.
- If the APTT is also prolonged, factor VIII/fibrinogen concentrate is recommended in addition to FFP.
- If none is available, give 10–15 units of ABO compatible cryoprecipitate, which contains factor VIII and fibrinogen.
- Give platelet concentrate (PCs) only when: (a) The patient shows clinical signs of microvascular bleeding, i.e., bleeding and oozing from mucous membranes, wounds, raw surfaces, and catheter sites. (b) The patient's platelet count falls below 50×10^9/L.
- Give sufficient PCs to stop microvascular bleeding and maintain an adequate platelet count.
- Consider PC transfusion in cases where the platelet count falls below 20×10^9/L, even if there is no clinical evidence of bleeding, because there is a danger of occult bleeding, such as into brain tissue. The prophylactic use of platelet concentrates in patients receiving large volume blood transfusions is not recommended.

Dilutional coagulopathy: Massive trauma causes hemorrhagic shock; in this condition, there is fluid shift from the interstitial to the intravascular compartment that leads to dilution of the coagulation factors and platelets. This is further accentuated when the lost blood is replaced with coagulation factor deficient fluids infusion of colloids and crystalloids induce coagulopathy to a greater extent than that explained by simple dilution.

Another cause is low **colloid oncotic pressure** giving rise to interstitial edema.

Transfusion of 500 mL of pRBC reduces clotting factor and platelet count by 10%.

Clinical effects are seen after 8 units PRBCs in adults.

10 units pRBC reduce platelet count by 50%.

Critical platelet level = 75,000 (i.e., 50%).

1 "dose" of platelets should increase count by 30,000/cu mm.

Each unit FFP should increase factors by 10%, but increase is only 2.5%.

Effect of Hypothermia: Incidence is 9% in trauma patients. Hypothermia is defined as a decrease in the core body temperature to <36 °C. The normal core body temperature in humans is maintained by the hypothalamus and typically ranges from 36.5 to 37.5 °C. Intraoperative hypothermia is associated with postoperative myocardial ischemia, impaired coagulation, an increased risk of wound infection, and atrioventricular arrhythmia. Massive blood infusion is one of the causes of hypothermia. One liter of fluid at room temperature will reduce the mean body temperature by approximately 0.25 °C. Induction of mild hypothermia without extracorporeal circulation, a 30-min infusion of 2 L of normal saline at 4 °C, decreases the core body temperature by 2.5 °C. At a temperature below 34 °C, there is slowing of enzyme activity and decreased platelet function. Hypothermia leads to decreased citrate metabolism and drug clearance and leads to the development of coagulopathy. Five units pRBC decrease temperature by 1 °C. Coagulopathy due to hypothermia is not reflected in laboratory tests as blood samples are warmed during processing.

ECG Changes in Hypothermia: An "Osborne wave" characterized by a notch in the downward portion of the R wave in the QRS complex and low-voltage bradycardia.

Mortality rate of hypothermia increases significantly if temperature <32 °C.

Prevention: The patient should always be kept warm, and blood warmer should be used when the infusion rate is above 50 mL/kg/h.

Effect of acidosis produces reduction in factor Xa/Va reduced.

Coagulation proteases optimum at pH 8.

Xa/Va complex activity reduced by 50% at pH 7.20, 70% at pH 7.0, and 90% at pH 6.8.

Base deficit predicts shock; shock predicts death. Base deficit of <6 can lead to 2% of patients with increased PTT and increased INR, and base deficit >6 are observed in 20% of patients with increased PTT/INR.

Box 10.7: Relation of pH and Reduction of Factor Xa/Va

pH	Factor Xa/Va reduced (%)
>7	50
7	70
<6.8	80

Calcium binding to factors decreases with acidosis (Box 10.7).

Hypocalcaemia: Blood and blood components pRBCs, fresh frozen plasma, and platelets contain citrate anticoagulant. Infusion of these blood components can lower plasma calcium level in patients and neonates.

ECG Changes in Hypocalcemia: The most significant sign is intermittent QT prolongation, or intermittent prolongation of the QTc (corrected QT interval) secondary to a lengthened ST segment.

Clinical symptoms of hypocalcemia include confusion; memory loss; muscle spasms; numbness; tingling in the hands, feet, and face; and depression.

Hyperkalemia: Stored blood contains high levels of potassium which, when infused, can be taken up by the red cells. The supernatant of stored RBCs usually contains more than 60 mEq/L of potassium. Potassium in stored blood increases due to decrease in ATP production and leakage of potassium into the supernatant. The potassium content decreases by warming of blood. It is ideal to use blood less than 10 days old and irradiated blood is more hypokalemic.

ECG Changes in Hyperkalemia: Tall, peaked T waves with a narrow base, best seen in precordial leads. Shortened QT interval and ST-segment depression.

Transfusion-associated hyperkalemic cardiac arrest is a serious complication in patients receiving packed red blood cell (pRBC) transfusions. Mortality from hyperkalemia increases with large volumes of pRBC transfusion, increased rate of transfusion, and the use of stored pRBCs. It is more marked in patients with renal failure and hypothermia or in neonates.

When a patient receives a massive transfusion of red cell products, hyperkalemia may occur if sufficiently large amounts of extracellular potassium are administered over a very short period. With the advent of high-capacity fluid warmers and large-caliber intravenous cannulas, more than four blood volumes (>40 units) can be transfused per hour. Thus, when using such devices, the rate of transfusion can be identified as an important factor in clinically significant complication.

Hypomagnesemia is an important electrolyte imbalance and in the massively transfused patient is most likely secondary to citrate toxicity is indicated by a low level of magnesium in the blood. The normal adult value for magnesium is 1.5–2.5 mEq/L.

ECG Changes in Hypomagenesemia: prolonged QTc. Atrial and ventricular ectopy, atrial tachyarrhythmia, and torsade's de pointes are seen in the.

Symptoms of Hypomagnesemia: It includes the development of muscle weakness, confusion, and decreased reflexes, "jerky" movements, high blood pressure, and irregular heart rhythms with severely low blood magnesium levels (Fig. 10.1).

Adult respiratory distress syndrome (ARDS): It can be due to under- and over-transfusion; the risk can be minimized by maintenance of good perfusion and oxygenation. When ARDS occurs during or following massive transfusion, transfusion-associated acute lung injury (TRALI) should be considered.

Massive transfusion protocol is not a blood product prescription. It is a pathway used to define when to initiate the protocol, what types of blood products to be released immediately, types of blood tests required in major bleeding episodes, assisting the interactions of the treating clinicians and the blood bank, and ensuring judicious use of blood and blood components and to activate arrangements for getting the blood products to the patient in short span of time.

Patients with ongoing or expected major bleeding would benefit from an accurate assessment of the functional state of the hemostatic system to provide optimal care, providing cost-effective replacement of only the needed blood components.

Maintaining blood in a liquid state is critical for homeostasis. It allows blood to supply an adequate delivery of oxygen and nutrients to tissues while also eliminating carbon dioxide and other waste products. On the other hand, the ability of blood to convert from a liquid to a solid state, in other words, to coagulate, underlies the mechanism that protects the body from life-threatening exsanguination. This process of thrombosis is normally a localized event at the site of vascular injury while the rest of the circulating blood remains in a liquid state.

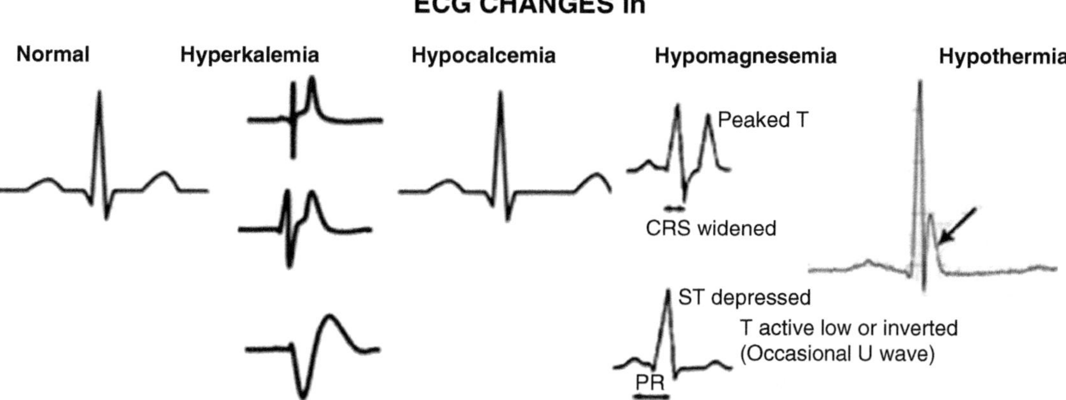

Fig. 10.1 ECG changes

10.4 Management of Loss of Blood Components

Blood component loss during massive blood loss is best managed by following the massive transfusion protocol (MTP). Mild to moderate blood loss can be managed with crystalloid or colloid infusions alone. However, with increasing loss, dilutional anemia and later dilutional coagulopathy set in.

MTPs are designed to interrupt the lethal triad of acidosis, hypothermia, and coagulopathy that develops with massive transfusion thereby improving outcome.

10.4.1 Steps in the Massive Hemorrhage Protocol

- **Step 1:** Early recognition of massive blood loss and triggering MTP based on clinical assessment.
- **Step 2:** Activate massive transfusion support protocol prescribe blood and blood products early to allow for delivery time lag and thawing time (30 min for FFP).
- Formula to assess which patients needs massive transfusion protocol (MTP)
- **Clinical judgment + Mechanism of injury + Pitfall conditions**
- It is important to identify early requirement of MTP and the logistics of how to administer it.
  1. If the patient is in an obvious shock state, or shock index is >1 or has an ABC score ≥2 activate the MTP.
  2. If none of these are present, consider the **resuscitation intensity in patients,** who require more than 4 units of any combination of crystalloids or blood products, to maintain adequate perfusion. The high resuscitation intensity predicts higher mortality, and an indication of MTP. Consider the patient's age, blood pressure medications, and baseline blood pressure in assessing for occult shock. Use clinical judgment, mechanism of injury, and pitfall conditions.
- **ABC score** 1 point for each of penetrating injury, positive FAST, SBP ≤90, and HR ≥120.
- A score of ≥2 indicates requirement for activation of MTP.
- Large volumes of crystalloid may lead to the "triangle of death"; goal should be to give crystalloid with cautions.
- **Pitfall conditions consider a lower threshold for activating MTP.**
- Patients taking anticoagulants and beta-blocker drugs for hypertension and elderly are not well represented in MTP studies and have a lower threshold for calling for blood transfusion needs.
- **Step 3:** Collect blood sample for crossmatch before any IV infusion as colloids infusion may interfere with cross matching (mainly dextrans by coating RBC surface).
- Prescribe inotrope and vasopressor drugs in established hypotension cases due to a blood loss to avoid critical hypoperfusion and to buy time for fluid resuscitation. They should be stopped as soon as volume deficits are replaced, and a safe blood pressure is achieved.
- Request shock pack issue (4 units of pRBC + 4 units of FFF), and prepare to issue 6 packs of pRBC + 6 packs of FFP.
- Do not exceed recommended maximum doses of colloid. Use of starch-based colloid solutions in large volumes in a hemodynamically critical patient is controversial in view of evidence of renal dysfunction associated with their use in intensive care unit.
- **Step 4:** Requirement for massive transfusion protocol support continues. Laboratory support to issue above +2x pools (of 5) cryoprecipitate, prepare to issue platelets 4 units.
- **Step 5:** Requirement for massive transfusion continues, and blood bank laboratory should actively manage blood and check and request resupply of appropriate.
- **Step 6:** Requirement for massive transfusion support continues, repeat step 5.

10.5 Trauma Transfusion: Order for Uncrossed Blood Components

- Patient's name
- Date of birth
- Patient's identity card number (Aadhar card)
- Hospital
- Surgeon Date of operation No of units required
- Unit number
- Serial number

Order	Transfuse blood product now	Order ID 001
Requested by	Dr	
Message: Notifies to the transfuge patient or his attendant in the event uncrossed blood product are transfuged, I accept responsibility for untoward transfusion reactions, which may have been prevented by routine compatibility testing.		
Performance date		
Priority	Stat	
Blood product	PRBCs	
Amount		
Measures	Units	
Transfuse over time		
Special procedure		
Consent obtained		
Recheck Hct order		
Special instructions		

Two categories of immediate life threats in trauma:

Massive external hemorrhage

Critical airway compromises:

Hypoxia (<90% oxygen saturation despite maximal noninvasive ventilation).

Dynamic airway (anticipates evolving disruption of airway, head and neck injuries that are expected to worsen over the next few minutes).

Once these two immediate life threats have been ruled out or managed, resuscitation should focus on hemodynamic optimization before definitive airway management.

Patient positioning in trauma: Avoid lying flat throughout the resuscitation.

Consider placing the trauma patient in reverse Trendelenburg immediately after the FAST exam to maximize respiratory physiology and CNS physiology, especially for the high BMI patient and/or the severely head-injured patient.

If a patient is more comfortable sitting up and/or refuses to lay flat, consider maintaining them in the sitting up position rather than laying them flat throughout the resuscitation. Forcing a patient to lay flat who is more comfortable sitting up may precipitate airway compromise.

The first and last 15 min of trauma management are critical for survival of trauma patients.

10.6 Occult Shock in Trauma Resuscitation

The early identification of occult shock is important because under-recognition is associated with worse patient outcomes.

10.6.1 How to Assess for Occult Shock in the First 15 min of Trauma Resuscitation

Calculate the **Shock Index (SI)**: heart rate (HR)/systolic blood pressure (SBP) if shock index >1 assume occult shock and implies a worse prognosis in 24 h after injury. Normal heart rate 60–80 min and normal systolic blood pressure 100–120 mmHg.

Assess the lowest BP measured and trend of BP over time; if isolated or persistent SBP <110, assume occult shock.

FAST positive with flat inferior vena cava.

Feel for the presence of peripheral pulses and look for signs of poorly perfused extremities.

Remember: Blood pressure and heart rate, when used individually, fail to accurately predict the severity of hypovolemia and shock in major trauma.

A single prehospital drop in BP may be a clue to impending catastrophic shock.

Record the most recent lowest BP.

10.6.2 Resuscitation Targets in the First 15 min of Trauma

There are two targets to be considered in early trauma resuscitation presumed to be caused by hemorrhagic shock.

Adequate tissue perfusion: presence of peripheral pulses in the blunt trauma patient, central pulses in the penetrating trauma patient.

Adequate hemostasis: While there are no evidence-based absolute BP targets in early trauma resuscitation that can be applied to all trauma patients, a reasonable guide is the following:

- **Presumed hemorrhagic shock**: Systolic BP <70 mmHg.
- **Presumed neurogenic shock**: If mean arterial pressure (MAP) is <60 mmHg. **MAP** ≥60 mmHg is believed to be needed to maintain adequate tissue perfusion. **MAP** ≥65 mmHg is recommended in patients with severe sepsis and septic **shock**.

Vasopressors are only indicated in presumed neurogenic shock in the setting of trauma.

10.6.3 Volume Resuscitation, Volume Challenge, Controlled Resuscitation, and Early Resuscitation Targets

Consider the following before volume resuscitation. The patient that is bleeding may not appear to be in shock, and the patient who is in shock may not be actively bleeding. It is imperative to identify active bleeding, obstructive shock, and neurogenic shock.

Large volumes of crystalloid contribute to the trauma "triangle of death" (metabolic acidosis, hypothermia, and coagulation derangements).

10.6.4 Initial Management

Initial resuscitation with replacement fluids (crystalloid (RL)—3 mL/mL of blood loss) is a priority to restore volume.

10.6.4.1 How to Give MTP

Give the MTP as 1:1:1 ratio of pRBCs, FFP, and platelet over the first 24 h. Give 4 units of red cells up front as they can usually be delivered faster that FFP and platelets.

In massive hemorrhage with shock, infusion rate of 40 mL/min (600 drops) per minute allows an entire unit of blood (400 mL) to be transfused in 10 min can be given and repeated. Infusion rate of 80 mL/min (1200 drops) are also required in dire emergency conditions and can be given; infusion rates of greater than 100 mL/min can lead to cardiac arrest.

10.7 Protocol of Supply of Blood Component in Massive Transfusion

Emergency: 2500 mL (50)% of blood volume with either whole blood of pRBC.

FFP, within 10 min.

Very urgent: 1500 mL (25)% blood within 15 min.

Urgent: 20% blood volume within 30 min.

Standby: 10–20% blood volume with in 1 h (Boxes 10.8 and 10.9).

10.7.1 Management of Intravascular Volume Loss

This is a vital component of blood loss management. Physiologically, hemodynamic compensatory mechanisms maintain vital organ perfusion till about 30% total blood volume loss, beyond

Box 10.8: Massive Transfusion Protocol in Hospital Practice

10 pRBC + 10 FFP + 2 platelets
Then 6 pRBC + 4 FFP + 2 platelets

Box 10.9: Current Battle Field Practice

10 pRBCs + 10 FFP + 10 platelets

which there is risk of critical hypoperfusion. Inadequate resuscitation at this stage leads to hemorrhagic shock. In case of over resuscitation leading to high arterial and venous pressures may be equally deleterious as it may dislodge hemostatic clots and cause more bleeding.

Massive transfusion protocols are activated by a clinician in response to massive bleeding. Generally this is activated after clinical judgment and need of massive transfusion during the course of treatment. MTPs have a predefined ratio of RBCs, FFP, and platelets units (random donor platelets) in each pack (e.g., 1:1:1 or 2:1:1 ratio) for transfusion. It is institution specific.

In patients with hemorrhagic shock, crystalloids and colloids are used for initial resuscitation. When blood and blood products become available, patients are transfused with required components.

10.7.2 Management of Massive Blood Loss by Pharmacological Support

Recombinant factor Vila (r FVila) is indicated in patients with hemophilia A and B for treatment of congenital factor VII deficiency.

It has the potential to reduce the need for massive transfusion in penetrating trauma. In addition, mortality may be reduced in blunt trauma. VIIa should be restricted to only when hemorrhage has not responded to transfusion or other conventional therapy (Box 10.10).

The recommended dose is 200 μg/kg initially followed by repeat dose of 100 μg/kg at 1 and 3 h.

Box 10.10: The Indications of Recombinant Factor Vila (r FVila)

Traumatic bleeding
Perioperative blood loss
Postpartum hemorrhage
Spontaneous intracerebral hemorrhage
Bleeding in liver diseases
Anticoagulant associated bleeding

Factor eighth inhibitor by pass activity (FEIBA) is an anti-inhibitor coagulant. Factor VIII complex is available in 500 U and& 1000 U powder and solvent for solution. It is indicated for use in hemophilia A and B patients with inhibitors for:

- Control and prevention of bleeding episodes.
- Perioperative management.
- Routine prophylaxis to prevent and to reduce the frequency of bleeding episodes.

FEIBA is not indicated for the treatment of bleeding episodes resulting from coagulation factor deficiencies in the absence of inhibitors to coagulation factor VIII or coagulation factor IX.

Tranexamic acid (TXA) (Beriplex) is an antifibrinolytic agent which has been shown to reduce overall mortality and death due to bleeding among severely injured patients when administered within the first 3 h following injury.

Indications:

1. Hemorrhage associated with trauma (consider use on all patients receiving blood products during initial resuscitation within 3 h of injury).
2. Hemorrhage or risk of hemorrhage in increased fibrinolysis or fibrinogenolysis

Contraindications: treatment given after 3 h after injury significantly increase the **risk of death**.

It is contraindicated in patients with DIC or uncompensated liver diseases.

10.7.3 Whole Blood or Blood Component in Obstetric Hemorrhage

Alexander et al., in an observational study of massive obstetric hemorrhage at Parkland hospital, showed whole blood to be superior to pRBCs or combined transfusions in preventing acute tubular necrosis and other complications. The availability of fresh warm blood in developing countries could provide an alternative to more expensive and infrastructure-dependent blood components. Whole blood replaces many coagulation factors, and its plasma expands blood volume. It has the added advantage of exposing the patient to fewer references.

Assessment of volume status in trauma: Vital signs are poor predictors of extent of bleeding. SVO_2 is a better predictor.

10.7.4 Limitations of Massive Transfusion Protocols

Not standardized: The trigger for initiating the protocol as well as the optimum ratio of pRBC/FFP/platelets is institution specific.

Wastage: If MTP is triggered for a non-massive blood loss situation, or the bleeding is controlled within short time, it may lead to wastage of blood products.

Associated problems secondary to volume resuscitation—They are:

- **Inadequate resuscitation:** Hypoperfusion leads to lactic acidosis, systemic inflammatory response syndrome (SIRS), disseminated intravascular coagulation and multiorgan dysfunction and failure. It also increases the expression of thrombomodulin on endothelium, which then complexes with thrombin, which in turn leads to a reduced amount of thrombin available to produce fibrin and increases the circulating concentrations of anticoagulant activated protein C, which worsens the coagulopathy.
- **Over resuscitation can lead to transfusion-associated circulatory overload (TACO):** This is a well-known condition that occurs due to large number of rapid transfusion of blood or blood products in a short time. This is most commonly seen in elderly patients, small children, and patients with compromised left ventricular function. Interstitial edema due to increased hydrostatic pressure can cause abdominal compartment syndrome.
- **Dilutional coagulopathy**: During hemorrhagic shock, there is fluid shift from the interstitial to the intravascular compartment that leads to dilution of the coagulation factors. This is further accentuated when the lost blood is replaced with coagulation factor deficient fluids. Studies have also shown that infusion of colloids and crystalloids may induce coagulopathy to a greater extent than that explained by simple dilution.
- Low colloid oncotic pressure giving rise to interstitial edema.

10.8 Measures for Control of Massive Bleeding

10.8.1 Vascular Access in the First 15 min of Trauma Resuscitation

Two short large bore peripheral IVs are recommended for initial vascular access in the trauma patient.

If a peripheral IV cannot be rapidly obtained, humerus intraosseous infusions (IO) with pressure bag have adequate infusion rates but should be used only as a bridge to venous access and should be checked frequently for flow.

A central line is mandatory for patients requiring long transport times or when resuscitative endovascular balloon occlusion of the aorta (REBOA) is planned even if two well running peripheral lines are established.

Intraosseous infusion (IO) is the process of injecting blood, fluids, or medicine directly into the marrow of a bone, when intravenous access is not available or not feasible. This provides a non-collapsible entry point into the systemic venous system in cases of trauma.

10.8.2 Resuscitative Endovascular Balloon Occlusion of the Aorta (REBOA)

Reboa is a technique used in trauma for patients that are rapidly bleeding to death from injuries to their chest, abdomen, or pelvis. This technique involves rapidly placing a flexible catheter into the femoral artery, maneuvering it into the aorta and inflating a balloon at its tip.

Large bore intravenous (IV) access: Two peripheral IV (14/16 G) cannulae or special wide bore cannulae (insertion sheath) can be put into the internal jugular vein. Fourteen gauge cannula gives flow rate of 250–300 mL/min and with 16 G flow rate of 150–240 mL can be achieved. Both are painful and require large insertions. In emergency situations, cannulation of external jugular vein may be considered. Eighteen gauge cannula gives flow rate of 100–120 mL/min and is most commonly used when the transfusion flow rate is moderately required. Twenty gauge provides flow rate of 55–80 mL/min and is used in older children, adolescent, and adult and is ideal for IV infusion and blood infusion at a slow rate. It is easy to insert into small, thin, fragile veins. Twenty-four gauge is used in infant, toddler, and older children and provides flow rate 23 mL/min.

Flow rate calculation: When calculating the flow rate of IV solutions, remember that the number of drops required to deliver 1 mL varies with the type of administration set.

$$\text{Flow rate} = \text{Volume of infusion in mL} \times \text{Drip factor}\left(\text{in drops / mL}\right) / \text{Time of infusion in minutes}$$

Types of Administration Sets

- Macrodrip set delivers (10–20 drops/mL)
- Microdrip set deliver (60 drops/mL)

Blood components: Blood components must be filtered with 170–260 micron filters to remove clots and small clumps of platelets and white blood cells that form during collection and storage.

Blood infusion: If more than 2 units are to be given consequently and they are ABO compatible with one another, one set may be used for both as long as they are infused within 4 h. Use new set for each component of blood component.

Leukocyte removal filter: they are different from red cell and platelet filters. Leukocyte filters are fixed with standard infusion set, and they are designed for gravity drip use and have special priming requirement.

IV pumps: Mechanical IV pumps are useful in children for controlling the slow infusion rate, but care is needed to avoid hemolysis.

Pressure bags are needed only in massive hemorrhage. The bag should be inflated only until the blood flow through the drip chamber is continuous, about 200 mmHg. Pressure of more than 300 mmHg may lyse the red cells and rupture of blood bag.

Blood warming devices: In-line fluid warmers and surface warmers **are** used to prevent cardiac arrhythmia associated with rapid infusion of large volume of cold blood.

Safest and the most common method of warming of blood is to pass through plastic coils or plastic cassettes in warm water 37–38 °C.

Adults receiving blood at a rate in excess of 100 mL/min.

Patient's with clinical significant cold agglutinins.

Rapid infusion of blood through central lines.

Blood warmer should have special software and monitor in-line devices.

Continuous core temperature monitoring.

Invasive arterial pressure monitoring.

Adequate amount of colloid (gelatins), crystalloid, infusion sets, and IV calcium preparations.

BLOOD WARMING DEVICES

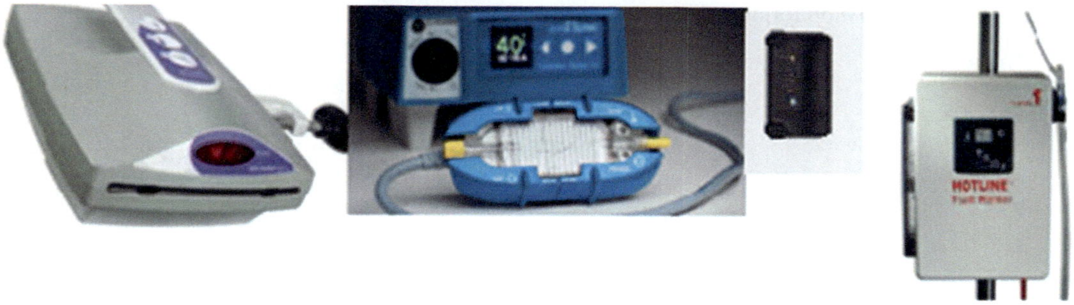

IV solutions and medications: 25 mL of normal saline can be infused before starting the blood transfusion. Dextrose may cause red cells to aggregate and lyse and, hence, not to be used. Ringer lactate may cause blood to clot due to the presence of calcium, hence not to be used. Never add drugs and medicines to blood bag.

EMIT HypothermX™ HX100 intravenous Blood & Fluid Warmer is a patent-protected portable fluid-warming device designed to warm intravenous fluids, blood, or blood products infused into a patient to prevent or treat trauma, environmental, procedure-related and/or procedure-induced hypothermia. Heating is accomplished via a flameless hydrocarbon combustion process fueled with a isobutane/propane mixture (Boxes 10.11 and 10.12).

Core temperature: Normal body temperature is measured by a thermometer placed in the mouth, the rectum, or the auditory canal (for tympanic membrane temperature). The normal oral temperature is 37 °C (98.6 °F); rectally, it is 37.3 °C (99.2 °F). The tympanic membrane temperature is a direct reflection of the body's core temperature.

The tympanic thermometer is a modern device that is attached to a handheld instrument and inserted into the inner ear; the blood flow in the vicinity of the tympanum, the middle ear, provides an accurate indication of the temperature at the body core.

Postoperative intensive care: Mechanical ventilation and continuous hemodynamic monitoring are usually required due to occurrence of circulatory overload and hemodynamics, biochemical instability, and invasive arterial pressure.

Invasive arterial pressure measurement allows beat-to-beat pressure measurement and has greater accuracy than cuff based measurements in low flow conditions. Also, the arterial catheter allows frequent arterial blood sampling which is useful in guiding therapy. Many modern hemodynamic monitors calculate pulse pressure variation which is a more specific indicator of volume responsiveness.

Role of central venous pressure monitoring: Central venous catheters, due to their length and high resistance, allow inferior flow rates than wide bore cannulae. However, they are useful for assessment of the hemodynamic status, administration of vasoactive agents and blood sampling (Box 10.13).

Laboratory values should be obtained frequently. The time lag between collection of samples and obtaining the reports is a serious limitation in their utility during rapid ongoing blood loss management.

Box 10.11: Point-of-Care Testing Is Extremely Important: Hourly, Are Useful in Directing Therapy

- Arterial blood gas (ABG)
- Hemoglobin (Hb)
- Thromboelastograph (TEG)
- Serum electrolytes
- Serum lactate levels

Box 10.12: Clinical Monitoring

- Electrocardiogram
- Capnometry
- Pulse oximetry
- Arterial blood pressure
- Core temperature
- Urine output

10.8.3 Role of Point-of-Care Coagulation Testing

An ideal test on blood coagulation does not yet exist. Coagulation tests usually have long processing times and may not be helpful in guiding

Box 10.13: Recommended Laboratory Test

- Hemoglobin
- Platelet count
- Prothrombin time (PT)
- Partial prothrombin time (aPTT)
- Ionized calcium
- ABG for acid–base status
- Central venous O_2 saturation/lactate as an indicator of tissue hypoperfusion

therapy in a rapid developing blood loss situation. However, results may be useful at a later stage to assess how the case developed.

Thromboelastography (TEG) is a noninvasive test that quantitatively measures the ability of whole blood to form a clot. The test is particularly very useful in severely injured person, liver transplant, cardiac surgery, and perioperative bleeding and for managing severe peripartum hemorrhage also rapid availability of results helps in timely intervention. TEG guide transfusion therapy and decrease the use of blood products. It has potential to deliver immediate goal-oriented and individualized care to a bleeding patient. It is a rapid real-time bedside test with a simple methodology (point-of-care testing).

Permissive hypotension is a fluid management strategy, often used in adult trauma settings, that targets a suboptimal arterial pressure until definitive management of bleeding can be obtained. It aims to maintain end-organ perfusion while limiting crystalloid resuscitation, thereby limiting dilutional coagulopathy, clot disruption, and cellular dysfunction.

10.8.4 Target Clinical and Laboratory End Point's Resuscitation in Massive Blood Loss

Mean arterial pressure (MAP) > 60 mmHg, systolic arterial pressure 80–100 mmHg (in hypertensive patients one may need to target higher MAP).

- Hb 7–9 g/dL
- INR <1.5
- Activated partial prothrombin time aPTT <42 s
- Fibrinogen >1.5–2 g/L
- Platelets >50 × 10^9/L
- pH 7.35–7.45
- Core temperature >35.0 °C
- Base deficit <3.0/L
- Serum lactates <2 mEq/L
- Urine output >40 mL/h
- CVP 0–5 mg
- PT and APTT ratio 1.5

Box 10.14: Types of Battle Field Injury

Blast wounds: Landmines, grenades, IEDs (improvised explosive device)
Suicide bombing
Amputation
Gunshot wounds and shrapnel wounds

10.9 Massive Blood Loss in Battle Field Injury

The modern battle field is more dangerous and violent than ever before. Primary blast injury is uncommon in most combat casualties but is considerably more common in casualties due to naval combat. The most common combat wounds include blast injury (Box 10.14).

Penetrating injuries are classified according to energy transferred—high, low, or mixed.

Mechanical and functional injuries: The effect of missile hitting any bone and fragments of bone may cause secondary injury. Shock waves may damage tissues remote from path of missile.

High energy wound: Causes temporary and permanent cavitation. Key features are size, shape, contamination, and clinical consequences.

War injury and need for blood: Over pressure affecting air containing organs—diffuse bleeding and non compressible hemorrhage.

Direct trauma: Traumatic amputations from flying objects and being thrown by blast, burns, and coagulopathies need for extensive debridement cutting back to healthy bleeding tissue.

10.9.1 Levels of Care

Military doctrine provides an integrated health support system, for triage (the assignment of degrees of urgency to wounds or illnesses to decide the order of treatment of a large number of patients or casualties), evacuation and treatment of the injured soldiers. In Armed Forces, there are five levels of care. They are:

- **Level 1** care is by self or buddy or at the remedial accomplishment plan (RAP).
- **Level 2** care is at Forward Surgical Centre or FSC of the field hospital meant for major life and limb saving surgery.
- **Level 3** is the highest care in the combat setting. It would mean treatment at a large general or zonal hospital.
- **Level 4** is treatment in command hospitals.
- **Level 5** is the highest care in civil or military superspeciality hospital.

Evacuation: Evacuation of casualty is done by air, motorized transport, or ambulances. Regional transfers are undertaken by train or fixed wing aircraft. Aircraft have revolutionized the rapid evacuation of casualties for definitive care, but in the Indian setup, ambulances, mules (domestic animals, like khacchar), and stretcher-bearers are still used in varying terrains and mountainous regions.

Three basic principles of treatment of wounded soldier: Enter, Evaluate, and Evacuate is a simple three-phase approach that guides the initial 30 min of a response to blast and active shooter events with causalities.

Field hospital is the "**emergency** hospital for the battle field," a **hospital** for the care and treatment of sick and wounded **military** personnel.

Intracorps medical regulating system: In this system, patients are transferred or forward support battalion evacuated from **main support battalion (MSB)** to a **combat support hospital (CSH).**

Intratheater medical regulating system: In this system, patients are transferred or evacuated from one hospital to another. This includes evacuation **emergency ambulatory care (EAC).**

Intertheater medical regulating system: moving patients between, into, and out of the different theaters of the geographic combatant commands.

Patient administrator: The patient administrator (PAD) accomplishes the medical regulating function at the hospital level in addition to his normal duties. His medical regulating functions include consolidating all evacuation requests within the hospital and forwarding an evacuation request to his next higher headquarters for action.

However, many developing countries and even some developed nations have not yet been able to present it in countries around the globe.

10.9.2 Type of Death in Battle Field Injury

The majority of deaths on the battle field today are non-survivable, defined as "any number of measures taken will not save the life of the severely wounded soldier."

1. However, among the group of potentially survivable fatalities, hemorrhage is the leading cause of death.
2. The resuscitation of patients with traumatic hemorrhagic shock is known as **damage control resuscitation (DCR)**.
3. The application of **DCR in the prehospital setting is termed remote damage control resuscitation (RDCR).**
4. Therapeutic options applied in RDCR can change as the challenges and timeline to reaching higher echelons of care are increased (e.g., military operations in far forward locations).

Golden hour container for collection and transportation of blood and components, designed for the extreme conditions of the military battle field, provides superior thermal protection for high value temperature-sensitive payloads between 2 and 96 L (plus cargo pallets too), from −50 °C to 25 °C for up to 7 days (168 h). The Golden Hour™ Medic Series 4 is a combat-portable pack that holds blood and other chilled medical supplies for 2 days in harsh conditions and up to 3 days in standard environments (Table 10.7).

Table 10.7 Shipment temperature protocol to reach at the site of treatment

Blood components	Temperature
Packed RBCs	1–10 °C
FFP	1–10 °C
Liquid plasma	1–10 °C
Platelet concentrate	Room temperature
Cryoprecipitate	1–10 °C

10.9.3 Treatment of War-Wounded Patients

Planning and prescreening are the most critical elements for successful **war blood bank donors (WBB).** Prescreened WBB donors are preferentially those currently on active duty, in the active reserve, or the active armed forces.

Aircraft carriers use a volunteer war blood bank registry that is routinely updated by a variety of scheduled events. A naval ship doctor in the preparation phase of deployment must enroll all the naval volunteers with details of medical information while at sea. A minimum of 300 registrants are maintained at all times by the ship's laboratory doctor-in-charge.

Local volunteer military donors: Requirements for blood products are ordinarily met through collection of donors in the volunteer military pool of all the forces including infantry, naval, air, and para-military forces by Armed Services blood donor centers. Eligible military donor pool categories are active duty (including BSF, coast guard, CRP, rapid action force, home guards and their dependents, and retirees and their dependents).

Military and para-military forces: to establish a memorandum of understanding (MOU) with local civilian blood banks or blood collection agencies for blood products when no other sources exist.

Walking blood bank program also known as pre-mission donated blood/field blood bank is a walking blood bank at the mission launch site that donates whole blood and stored refrigerated at 2–6 °C. The military unit then brings stored whole blood on specific missions in golden hour container to ensure temperature stability. The following things should be taken into consideration:

1. Prescreen your unit prior to deployment.
2. Keep a roster of personnel that are co-located with you like cooks, mechanics, para-engineers, porters, washerman, and likewise.

Blood training program: All unit personnel must attend a 1-week training program and refresher courses for resuscitation, how to treat life-threating hemorrhagic shock, blood typing, and crossmatching. In general, it spreads awareness of this procedure and its possible complications, since this technique is a perishable skill and it requires repeat courses again and again.

10.9.4 Detection of Blood Group at the War Site by Eldon Card

There are two types of kits designed for military use: (1) the one-man kit designed for the individual soldier to use in the field and secure him and (2) the military kit designed for field hospitals; a large number of tests can be performed from one kit.

10.9.4.1 Principle of Eldon Card

The Eldon card has four circles with antibody reagents. These antibodies will agglutinate with the corresponding antigens, if a person has the antigen in his blood. When a drop of blood is added in all the four circles, some of them will show agglutination depending on the blood group of the person according to which antibody field react and start agglutinating, and in the guide which comes with the Eldon blood type test, you can see which blood type you have according to which antibody fields react.

10.9.5 Advantages of the Eldon Card

Exceptionally easy to use, erase all human error, card can be kept in pocket, portable and compact, results ready in 2–5 min, blood can be grouped outside the blood bank, e.g., at the bedside just prior to a transfusion, in the practitioner's clinic, on remote locations as ships and oil rigs, on the battle field, in the class room, in the private home, or in any emergency situation calling for a speedy and reliable test. There is no need for refrigeration or electricity, and the test is stable and accurate in all locations. The only thing needed is a small amount of water in drinking quality.

10.9.6 Procedure

1. Activate the serum on the circles by adding a drop of water.
2. Sterilize finger with spirit or alcohol pad, and use a lancet to prick finger. Massage finger to get a free flow of blood.
3. Use a plastic Eldon stick to transfer the blood to the serum and stir the blood.
4. Use a new stick for each test circle to prevent cross-contamination.
5. Slowly tilting the card will prevent coagulation while the antibodies react to the serum on the card. Presence of clumping is positive test.
6. Clean finger with alcohol pad and apply a bandage.

Do NOT touch anyone else's blood. Throw all materials into the biohazard container.

10.9.7 How to Read Eldon Card

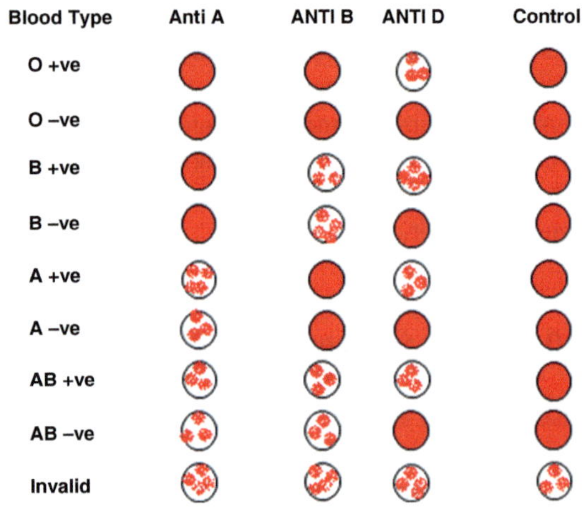

Blood Type Anti A ANTI B ANTI D Control
O +ve
O −ve
B +ve
B −ve
A +ve
A −ve
AB +ve
AB −ve
Invalid

Management of battle field blood transfusion: The leading cause of death on the battle field is uncontrolled hemorrhage. Military personnel are highly exposed to austere environmental conditions. In this setting **fresh whole blood** and **cold stored whole blood** is used in the treatment of exsanguinating hemorrhage. No current evacuation system, military or civilian, is capable of providing fresh whole blood and blood components in a prehospital environment, especially in austere settings. As a result, for the vast minority of casualties, in austere settings, with life-threatening hemorrhage, it is appropriate to consider a whole blood-based resuscitation approach to provide a balanced response to altered hemostasis and oxygen debt with the goal of reducing the risk of death from hemorrhagic shock. The use of fresh whole blood (FWB) in the civilian sector is far less established because of the availability of fractionated components, which mimic whole blood when given in a 1:1:1 ratio. Access to these components requires a robust supply chain that is vulnerable to disruption via terrorist attack and natural disaster.

Definition of warm whole blood (WHB), cold whole blood (CWB), and **Fresh blood (FB):** Warm whole blood is the fresh blood which is maintained at 22–27 °C after donation; if the donated blood is cooled to 2–6 °C, it is called as cold whole blood. Whole blood stored for less than 48 h is referred to as "fresh."

Red cells, plasma, and platelets are needed for clot formation. Consideration of these facts leads to the conclusion that whole blood should be transfused in situations of life-threatening hemorrhage, particularly when standard blood components are unavailable.

Field blood transfusion kit: Designed for field forward missions in the most remote and austere environments, it contains essential items to collect and transfuse fresh whole blood in a compact package.

The use of fresh whole blood in military settings is reserved for casualties who are anticipated to require massive transfusion (≥10 units

RBCs in 24 h) or have clinically significant shock despite optimal component therapy (i.e., apheresis platelets and FFP).

Buddy transfusion: Military person on the scene draw 1 unit of blood from a fellow soldier and subsequently administer it to the wounded soldier after making ABO and Rh (D) group by Eldon card test.

Damage control resuscitation: Aim is to establish early surgical control of bleeding.

- To prevent and/or treat acidosis, hypothermia, hypocalcaemia, coagulopathy, and shock.
- The battleship premise of first "patching up the holes," and delaying definitive care.
- Contraindicated in traumatic brain injury.

Hemostatic resuscitation considerations: To prevent or treat coagulopathy of trauma.

- 1:1:1 ratio of FFP/pRBC/platelet.
- Use of Thawed Plasma.
- Limit excessive use of pRBCs and crystalloids to prevent dilutional coagulopathy.
- Use of pRBCs of Decreased Storage Age.
- Consider early use of fibrinogen (Cryo) and rFVIIa.
- Warm fresh whole blood: when available.

Further Reading

Bolliger D, Görlinger K, Tanaka KA. Pathophysiology and treatment of coagulopathy in massive hemorrhage and hemodilution. Anesthesiology. 2010;113(5):1205–19.

Calvert C, Thomas SL, Ronsmans C, Wagner KS, Adler AJ, Filippi V. Identifying regional variation in the prevalence of postpartum haemorrhage: a systematic review and meta-analysis. PLoS One. 2012;7(7):e41114.

Calvert C, Thomas SL, Ronsmans C, et al. Identifying regional variation in the prevalence of postpartum haemorrhage: a systematic review and meta-analysis. PLoS One. 2012;7:e41114.

Cherkas D. Traumatic hemorrhagic shock: advances in fluid management. Emerg Med Pract. 2011;13(11):1–9.

Chidester SJ, Williams N, Wang W, Groner JI. A pediatric massive transfusion protocol. J Trauma Acute Care Surg. 2012;73(5):1273–7.

Dutton RP. Pathophysiology of traumatic shock. Semin Anesth Periop Med Pain. 2001;20(1):7–10.

Hockberger RS. Rosen's emergency medicine concepts and clinical practice. Philadelphia, PA: Elsevier, Inc.; 2018.

National Institute for Health and Care Excellence. Major trauma: assessment and initial management. NICE guideline [NG 39]; 2016.

Nunez TC, Young PP, Holcomb JB, Cotton BA. Creation, implementation, and maturation of a massive transfusion protocol for the exsanguinating trauma patient. J Trauma. 2010;68(6):1498.

O'Keeffe T, Refaai M, Tchorz K, Forestner JE, Sarode R. A massive transfusion protocol to decrease blood component use and costs. Arch Surg. 2008;143(7):686–91.

Perel P, Roberts I. Colloids versus crystalloids for fluid resuscitation in critically ill patients. Cochrane Database Syst Rev. 2012;(6):CD000567.

Rath WH. Postpartum hemorrhage–update on problems of definitions and diagnosis. Acta Obstet Gynecol Scand. 2011;90(5):421–8.

Riskin DJ, Tsai TC, Riskin L, Hernandez-Boussard T, Purtill M, Maggio PM, Spain DA, Brundage SI. Massive transfusion protocols: the role of aggressive resuscitation versus product ratio in mortality reduction. J Am Coll Surg. 2009;209(2):198–205.

Scharte M, Fink MP. Red blood cell physiology in critical illness. Crit Care Med. 2003;31(12):S651–7.

Sihler KC, Napolitano LM. Complications of massive transfusion. Chest. 2010;137(1):209–20.

Solomon C, Collis RE, Collins PW. Haemostatic monitoring during postpartum haemorrhage and implications for management. Br J Anaesth. 2012;109(6):851–63.

Spinella PC, Cap AP. Whole blood: back to the future. Curr Opin Hematol. 2016;23(6):536–42.

11 Autologous Blood Transfusion

11.1 Autologous Blood Transfusion (ABT)

Autologous blood transfusion (ABT) can be defined as a procedure in which blood is taken from a donor prior to need and returned to his circulation at some later time. Autologous transfusion can be performed in four ways:

1. Preoperative blood collection (POBD) (7–30 days), storage, and retransfusion during surgery.
2. Immediate preoperative phlebotomy with subsequent artificial hemodilution by crystalloids and later return of the phlebotomized blood. It is also known as an acute normovolemic hemodilution (ANH).
3. Intraoperative blood salvage and retransfusion.
4. Postoperative collection: Blood is collected from the drainage devices and reinfused to the patient.

All four methods of autologous transfusion offer an alternative method of blood transfusion in selected group of patients which eliminates many of the problems and complications associated with the banking and administration of homologous donor blood.

History of autologous blood transfusion: Reinfusion of blood was employed as early as 1818, and preoperative donation was advocated in the 1930s.

Blood salvaging was reported during neurosurgical and obstetric procedures from 1936.

Technologic advances made possible the development of safe, easy to use devices for recovery and reinfusion of shed blood.

Fear of transmitted diseases by allogeneic blood donor stimulated the growth of autologous program.

Criteria for autologous donors can be considered before any elective surgical procedures where a significant blood loss is expected (especially in POBD). There are no age limits for autologous donors. The minimum weight requirement for autologous donors is 50 kg (110 lb). Before the first donation, donors must have minimum hemoglobin of 11 g% and a minimum hematocrit of 33%. At subsequent donations, the minimum hemoglobin required is 10.5 g% with a minimum hematocrit of 32%.

Those with lesser body weight can donate proportionately lesser volume. Adolescents, children below 10 years, and the elderly also can be a candidate and can safely donate.

P. S. Ajmani, *Immunohematology and Blood banking*, https://doi.org/10.1007/978-981-15-8435-0_11

11.1.1 Time for Preoperative Blood Donation

Predonation usually begins 4 weeks prior to the anticipated need, depending on the number of units required.

Usually one donation per week is done. In 4 weeks we can have 4 units of blood.

If donor selection and procedure are appropriate, complications are very rare.

Vasovagal reactions may occur in female, and appropriate precautions are mandatory.

Time interval between the last donation and the surgery should be more than 72 h.

To prevent anemia due to donations, hematinic are prescribed 2 months before donation of first blood.

Use of recombinant erythropoietin is indicated to increase red cell production above the physiological level so that more blood units could be donated in a short span of time. It takes 3 days to detect a reticulocyte response and at least 10–14 days for any significant rise in hemoglobin. Both intravenous and subcutaneous administrations are commonly used to deliver RHuEPO. Subcutaneous administration is more convenient as it does not require any venous access. When compared with the intravenous route, subcutaneous RHuEPO administration significantly prolongs the increase of serum erythropoietin, thus sustaining the stimulation of erythropoiesis.

11.1.2 Protocol for Autologous Blood Bag

It must be labeled with sticker as "Autologous blood."

If any testing is reactive on a current collection or within the last 30 days, it must also be labeled "Biohazard."

Untested autologous units must be labeled "Donor Untested."

If the blood tested negative within the last 30 days, it must be labeled "Donor Tested within the last 30 days."

The donations must be processed and tested in the same way as donor blood and are subject to the same requirements for traceability.

Autologous blood will be discarded at outdate (35 days after donation) unless the blood bank is notified (before outdate) of extended surgery date.

11.2 Indication of Autologous Blood Transfusion

Patients with rare blood group or multiple blood group antibodies where compatible allogeneic (donor) blood is difficult to obtain.

Patients who are prone to development of serious psychiatric risk, if exposed to donor blood.

Children undergoing major surgeries like scoliosis

.

Patients who do not accept donor blood transfusions but are prepared to accept and consent to autologous blood.

When blood loss of more than 20% of blood volume in elective and emergency surgery. They are cardiovascular surgery, liver transplantation, neurosurgery, radical prostatectomy, orthopedic surgery, and gynecology operations.

11.2.1 Absolute Contraindication of Autologous Blood Transfusion

Idiopathic hypertrophic sub-aortic stenosis
Aortic stenosis
Left main coronary artery disease
Unstable angina
Myocardial infarction with 6 weeks of a donation date
Atrioventricular block
Evidence of infection or risk of bacteremia such as indwelling urinary catheter

11.2.2 Relative Contraindication

Untreated hypertension.
Coagulation disorder.

11.3 Advantages of Autologous Blood Transfusion

Provides fresh autologous blood product compared to stored blood. It has functional platelets; normal levels of clotting factors and 2,3-DPG; and no biochemical alterations associated with storage.

It is the least expensive method of autologous blood procurement.

It decreases the risk of transfusion reaction due to blood administration error.

Eliminates the risk of infection transmission associated with volunteer donor blood.

Eliminates the risk of allergic and acute hemolytic transfusion reactions.

Avoidance of immunosuppressive effects of allogenic transfusion.

11.4 Autologous Transfusion Options

11.4.1 Preoperative Blood Collection (POBD)

POBD refers to the donation of blood by a patient for his/her own future use; generally this is for a scheduled elective surgery. Blood is collected and stored prior to anticipate need. The top indications for preoperative blood donation (POBD) are total hip replacement, total knee replacement, hysterectomy, and major surgeries requiring more than 3 units of blood. POBD is most beneficial in procedures with substantial anticipated blood loss such as vascular and cardiothoracic surgery. Autologous collection should be considered only if the chance of requiring a transfusion exceeds 10% of total blood volume. Patients with low-risk surgeries that rarely require blood should not be considered for a POBD.

Table 11.1 Technique of preoperative blood donation method (leap and frog method)

Step	Day	Draw	Replace	Reserve	Net loss
I	0	1 unit A	None	Unit A	1 unit
II	7	Units B and C	Unit A	Unit B and C	2 units
III	14	Unit D and E	Unit B	Unit C, D, and E	3 units
IV	21	Unit F and G	Unit C	Unit D, E, F, G	4 units

11.4.2 Number of Autologous Blood Donations

The majority of autologous donors donate one or two donations depending on the type of surgery or treatment required. A maximum of four donations can be collected from the patient. The donations are normally drawn 1 week apart. Most healthy adult patients can donate up to 4 red cell units before elective surgery (Table 11.1).

On day 28 units D and E (2 weeks old) and F and G (1 week old) are available (total 4 units) which can be given to the patients when needed.

Perioperative collection and administration also known as acute normovolemic hemodilution (ANH): Blood is collected at the start of surgery and then infused during or after the procedure.

Intraoperative collection: Shed blood is recovered from the surgical field and transfused after decontamination of blood.

Postoperative collection: Blood is collected from the drainage devices and reinfused to the patient.

11.4.2.1 Perioperative Collection or Acute Normovolemic Hemodilution (ANH)

Definition: It is the removal of blood from a patient just before surgery and transfused immediately after surgery. In ANH 1–2 units of blood are collected into standard blood donation packs immediately before surgery (usually in the operation theater), and the patient's blood volume is maintained by the simultaneous infusion of crystalloid or colloid fluids. The blood is stored in the operation theater at room temperature and reinfused at the end of surgery or if significant bleeding occurs during surgery. ANH is most often used in cardiac bypass surgery where the immediate postoperative transfusion of "fresh whole blood" containing platelets and clotting factors is seen as an advantage.

Physiological changes in ANH which occurs in patient's body: Withdrawal of whole blood (in standard blood bag) and replacement with crystalloids and colloids result into sudden drop in Hct and arterial oxygen content, decreased blood viscosity, and increased cardiac output and peripheral resistance, and oxygen delivery to tissue is not affected; heart rate, CVP, and blood pressure remain unchanged.

Advantages of ANH: ANH is simple and less expensive than other techniques and provides fresh whole blood for transfusion.

No biochemical alterations associated with storage.

There is no hypothermia because the infused blood is kept at room temperature.

Platelet function is preserved, and there is no reduction in oxygen-carrying capacity of RBC.

RBC loss during surgery is less because it is diluted with fluid infused. Hemodilution decreases blood viscosity, which improves tissue perfusion; it is possible for emergency surgeries.

ANH complications: There is an acute and significant reduction in hematocrit leading to hemodynamic instability and a possibility of myocardial ischemia in susceptible patients.

11.4.2.2 Intraoperative Cell Salvage (ICS)

This is the collection and reinfusion of blood spilled during surgery.

ICS is now widely used in women at high risk of postpartum hemorrhage during cesarean section and in the management of major obstetric hemorrhage.

Commercially available, largely automated devices are available for ICS and are now widely used in hospitals for both elective and emergency surgery with significant blood loss and in the management of major traumatic or obstetric hemorrhage. The machines must always be used and maintained according to the manufacturer's instructions by appropriately trained staff. Blood lost into the surgical field is filtered to remove particulate matter and aspirated into a collection reservoir where it is anticoagulated with heparin or citrate. If sufficient blood is collected and the patient requires transfusion, the salvaged blood can be centrifuged and washed in a closed, automated system. Red cells suspended in sterile saline solution are produced, which must be transfused to the patient within 4 h of processing.

The reinfusion bag should be labelled in the operating theater with the minimum patient identifiers derived from the patient's ID band. The red cells are transfused through a 200 μm screen filter, as in a standard blood administration set, except in those instances where a leucodepletion filter is indicated. The transfusion should be prescribed and documented, and the patient monitored in the same way as for any transfusion.

Intraoperative Cell Salvage (ICS) Contraindication

IICS should not be used when bowel contents contaminate the operation site, and blood should not be aspirated from bacterially infected surgical fields.

Because of concerns about cancer cell reinfusion and spread, manufacturers do not recommend ICS in patients having surgery for malignant disease and peritonitis.

11.4.2.3 Postoperative Cell Salvage (PCS)

PCS is mainly used in orthopedic procedures, especially after knee or hip replacement and in correction of scoliosis. Blood is collected from wound drains and from cavities (such as a joint space into which bleeding has occurred) and returned through a filter which removes big items (like thrombi and tissue fragments) and other debris but does not remove inflammatory chemical mediators and then either filtered or washed in an automated system before reinfusion to the patient.

The simple filtration systems for reinfusion of washed red cells are mainly used when expected blood losses are between 500 and 1000 mL. With these infusion volumes, concerns about adverse effects on blood coagulation have not been confirmed in routine practice. Clinical staff must be trained, and competency assessed to use the device, accurately document the collection, and label the pack at the bedside. Collection of salvaged blood must be completed within the manufacturer's specified time (usually 6 h), and the reinfusion must be monitored and documented in the same way as donor transfusions.

PCS is relatively cheap and has the potential to reduce exposure to donor blood. It remains unclear whether it adds significantly to a comprehensive blood conservation program which includes preoperative optimization of Hb, hemostatic/antifibrinolytic measures during surgery, and strict postoperative transfusion thresholds.

Salvage can be one of the most expensive autologous techniques because costly capital equipment and disposables are used, and it is usually restricted to procedures resulting in substantial blood loss (>1–2 L), for example, cardiac surgery, trauma surgery, and liver transplantation.

Contraindications for postoperative cell salvage (PCS): Presence of bacterial infection or suspicion of malignant cells in the operative field and microfibrillar collagen or other foreign material at the operative site.

11.4.3 Characteristics of Processed Intra- and Postoperative Blood by Cell Saver

The characteristics of this type of blood are as follows:

- **HCT** of processed blood is 50–60% and can be varied by altering the processing parameters.
- Oxygen transport properties and survival of RBCs are equal or superior to stored allogeneic blood.
- Processed blood has a high 2,3-DPG level.
- pH of salvaged blood is alkaline (Box 11.1).

Box 11.1: Complications of Intra- and Postoperative Blood Salvaging

Air embolism
Fat embolism
Sepsis
A renal dysfunction due to free Hb and fragmented RBCs

11.5 Factors Determining Efficacy of Hemodilution

Initial hematocrit: Patients with higher hematocrits are able to provide more red cells for storage prior to the operation. The patient's beginning hematocrit and blood volume are key factors in estimating the amount of blood that should be removed prior to surgery.

Blood volume: Blood volume increases with weight. The "ideal" 70 kg male has approximately a 5 L of blood volume. Females have a slightly lower blood volume on a weight basis. For example, a 55 kg, adolescent female's blood volume would be approximately 3500 mL (55 kg × 60–65 mL/kg).

Intraoperative blood loss: The most obvious main determinant of red cell loss is blood loss during the operation.

Intraoperative management: If normovolemia is not effectively reestablished and maintained following removal of the autologous blood, then the procedure offers no benefit in terms of reducing red cell losses. In the absence of hemodilution, operative blood loss would occur at the higher preoperative hematocrit level.

The timing of red cell replacement is another factor that influences the effectiveness of ANH. When the stored blood is replaced after the operative blood loss, then the patient will experience the least red cell losses. From a safety perspective, occasionally, blood removed prior to operation may need to be transfused to treat severe anemia during the operation.

11.6 Reasons of Decreasing Autologous Blood Transfusion

The reasons for the observed decrease in autologous blood component collection and use include advances in surgical techniques, patient blood management (PBM) programs, and a decreasing risk of transfusion-transmitted infections with allogeneic blood.

Further Reading

AuBuchon JP, Popovsky MA. The safety of preoperative autologous blood donation in the nonhospital setting. Transfusion. 1991;31(6):513–7.

British Committee for Standards in Haematology, Transfusion Task Force, Boulton FE, James V. Guidelines for policies on alternatives to allogeneic blood transfusion. 1. Predeposit autologous blood donation and transfusion. Transfus Med. 2007;17(5):354–65.

Cohen JA, Brecher ME. Preoperative autologous blood donation: benefit or detriment? A mathematical analysis. Transfusion. 1995;35(8):640–4.

Goodnough LT. Blood and blood conservation: a national perspective. J Cardiothorac Vasc Anesth. 2004;18(4):S6–11.

Goodnough LT, Brecher ME, Kanter MH, AuBuchon JP. Transfusion medicine—blood transfusion. N Engl J Med. 1999;340(6):438–47.

Goodnough LT, Shander A, Spence R. Bloodless medicine: clinical care without allogeneic blood transfusion. Transfusion. 2003;43(5):668–76.

Hillyer CD, Silberstein LE, Ness PM, Anderson KC, Roback JD. Blood banking and transfusion medicine E-Book: Basic principles and practice. Philadelphia, PA: Elsevier Health Sciences; 2006.

Hutton D. SI03 the Standing Advisory Committee on Care and Selection of Donors. Transfus Med. 2006;16:3.

Kilduffe RA, DeBakey ME. The blood bank and the technique and therapeutics of transfusions. St. Louis: CV Mosby Company; 1942.

Mann M, Sacks HJ, Goldfinger D. Safety of autologous blood donation prior to elective surgery for a variety of potentially "high-risk" patients. Transfusion. 1983;23(3):229–32.

National Blood Resource Education Program (US). Use of autologous blood. Bethesda, MD: National Heart, Lung, and Blood Institute; 1994.

Spiess BD, Sassetti R, McCarthy RJ, Narbone RF, Tuman KJ, Ivankovich AD. Autologous blood donation: hemodynamics in a high-risk patient population. Transfusion. 1992;32(1):17–22.

Thomas MG, Gillon J, Desmond MJ. Preoperative autologous donation. Transfusion (Philadelphia, PA). 1996;36(7):633–9.

Blood Management 12

12.1 Patient Blood Management (PBM)

Blood transfusion is one of the most frequently used therapies worldwide and is associated with benefits, risks, and costs**. Blood transfusion is a liquid organ transplant**. PBM established 10 clinical recommendations and 12 research recommendations for preoperative anemia, RBC transfusion thresholds for adults, and implementation of PBM programs. PBM puts the patient at the heart of decisions made about blood transfusion to ensure they receive the best treatment and avoidable; inappropriate use of blood and blood components is reduced **in an effort to improve patient outcome.** Blood use in adult patients undergoing elective surgery demonstrated three main predictors for red blood cell transfusions:

Preoperative anemia, volume of surgical blood loss, and failure to adopt a more restrictive threshold for transfusion.

An increasing focus on PBM has been driven by a number of factors including:

- The risks associated with blood transfusion.
- With increasing evidence of increased length of stay and higher risk of morbidity and mortality.
- Rising healthcare costs to hospitalized patient both direct and indirect.
- Challenges of maintaining an adequate blood supply in the face of increased demand.

Patient blood management if properly implemented benefitted by:
- Increased patient satisfaction.
- Decrease the need for transfusion.
- Improved patient outcomes.
- Healthcare cost savings.

Hospital-based policy should be that every drop of blood counts. PBM represents an international initiative in best practice for transfusion medicine. Previous initiatives to reduce red cell usage have been very successful. Through sharing data on blood usage, providing examples of best practice and overcoming barriers to change, it will be possible to reduce further inappropriate use of all blood components. Healthcare costs are increasing faster than any other thing all over the world. Enhanced quality control in blood ensures the safest possible product but at increased cost. As new threats to the blood supply are discovered, more and more tests are required on every unit of blood resulting in increased cost of blood products. Cost includes collection, storage, and testing blood samples with safety checks at every step.

Stakeholders: Everyone involved in blood transfusion needs to take responsibility for

P. S. Ajmani, *Immunohematology and Blood banking*, https://doi.org/10.1007/978-981-15-8435-0_12

ensuring it is used appropriately. PBM needs leadership and support at every level, from national and regional leaders to trust management, health professionals, and their colleagues within the hospitals.

12.2 Benefits of Patient Blood Management

12.2.1 Patient Benefit

Blood components are used to save and improve millions of lives each year. The risk of serious complications of a blood transfusion is very low, but patients should only receive blood they really need.

12.2.2 Sustainability of the Blood Supply

While the overall demand for red cells is increasing year on year, the demand for platelets is more marked and may be due to factors such as medical advances and an aging population. Only 4.5% of the eligible population give blood, and new donors are always needed to replace regular donors who can no longer donate.

12.2.3 Use of Strict Transfusion Triggers

All blood products are transfused when the patient's laboratory values fall below a threshold. Using these triggers has markedly reduced the frequency of transfusion. A restrictive strategy (<7 g/dL) of packed red cell transfusion is at least as effective as and possibly superior to a transfusion strategy. Sometimes, several blood management strategies are used at the same time to avoid blood transfusion. No single approach (drug, device, technique) is effective for every patient (Boxes 12.1 and 12.2).

Box 12.1: The Three Pillars of Patient Blood Management (PBM)

Patient centered decision-making
Detection and management of anemia
Minimization of bleeding and blood loss

Box 12.2: Patient-Centered Decision-Making: Provide Verbal and Written Information to Patients Who May have a Transfusion, Explaining

The reason for transfusion
The risks and benefits
The transfusion process
Specific transfusion need
Alternatives to transfusion
That they are encouraged questions

12.3 Managing Anemia

Make an early diagnosis ongoing anemia and its causes, contributing factors and apply evidence-based rationale for use of red cells. Patients who are having an elective surgery procedure with a risk of blood loss are identified and assessed 4 weeks prior to surgery. Allows sufficient time to diagnose and manage anemia to avoid risk of transfusion.

12.3.1 Optimizing Coagulation

Evaluate both qualitative and quantitative measures to assess coagulation status.

Accurately assess cause of dysfunctional bleeding.

Employ goal directed therapy to correct coagulation abnormalities.

Apply evidence-based rationale for use of plasma.

Strategies to accurately assess the cause of bleeding dysfunction.

Rapid identification of coagulation abnormalities by point-of-care (POC) testing.

Use of platelet function testing such as thromboelastometry helps in timely decision to control bleeding.

12.3.2 Preoperative Assessment and Management

Preoperative risk stratification is important. A bleeding history should be obtained asking about past history of bleeding after surgery or trauma, childbirth, and menorrhagia in females, family history of bleeding diathesis and medication history particularly related to anticoagulants. The type of surgical intervention should also be considered with respect to the risk of bleeding, and meticulous planning is required by the perioperative surgical team.

12.3.3 Intraoperative

Intraoperative management of blood loss may be influenced by surgical technique, anesthetic blood loss reduction strategies, and pharmacological management.

Surgical technique is the key factor in determining perioperative blood loss. Minimally invasive surgery such as laparoscopic, robot-assisted, and endovascular techniques are associated with a reduction in blood loss when compared with open more invasive procedures.

12.4 Practical Implementation of Patient Blood Management (PBM)

Patient blood management program is a team approach. All hospitals should have a hospital transfusion committee (HTC) to decide wide blood conservation policy and protocols, continuing education for physicians, nurses, community, and patient education under leadership of physician and expertise in blood bank technology and advancement. Greater staff education and engagement can subsequently improve the education and engagement of patients with respect to the risks and benefits of blood transfusion.

Bench marking of performance including transfusion rates can help to identify particular areas of need, while preparation of business cases for PBM initiatives require management backing. Data collection and audit of progress is essential to the continued success of such initiatives. Parameters which should be monitored include:

- Use of blood components against local and national guidelines.
- Proportions of blood components transfused with pretransfusion blood results.
- Clinical indication documentation: proportion of preoperative patients screened for anemia before surgery where blood transfusion is most likely.

12.5 Advantages of Blood Conservative Program

- Responsive to public concern over safety of blood transfusion and its products.
- It sustains the blood supply.
- It improve technology, devices, and drugs.
- It is imperative to reducing hospital costs.
- It improves physician skills and improves patient care.
- It gives recognition as a "best practices" hospital and hospital stay on top in competitive time.

Further Reading

National Blood Authority Patient Blood Management Guidelines. Module 1 – Critical bleeding/massive transfusion, Australia; 2011.

National Health and Medical Research Council (NHMRC). A guide to the development, implementation and evaluation of clinical practice guidelines, Australia; 1999.

NHMRC/Australasian Society of Blood Transfusion (ASBT). Clinical practice guidelines on the use of blood components, Australia; 2001.

Society for the Advancement of Blood Management. Professional definition Patient Blood Management. [cited 2012 September 11]. Available from: http://www.sabm.org/.

Thomson A, Farmer S, Hofmann A, Isbister J, Shander A. Patient Blood Management - a new paradigm for transfusion medicine? ISBT Sci Ser. 2009;4(n2):423–35.

13 Blood Bank Protocols

All requests for blood or blood products and all blood bank diagnostic tests should be submitted on the blood bank requisition.

13.1 Blood Bank Requisition Form

Name of the hospital
Address
Phone number
E-mail address
Blood bank hours:
Routine Service: Monday–Saturday 8 AM–5 PM
Emergency (STAT) service: 24 hours all the 7 days
Telephone number of blood bank
Mobile number
Type of request (planned, urgent, rush)
Date and time received
Name of the patient — Age and sex
Family name of the patient — First name:
Address
Blood group
Rh (D) group
Patient IPD number
Ward number/nursing home
Name and signature of blood drawer
Time and date of blood taken
Indication of blood transfusion
History of previous blood component therapy
History of blood reactions if any
History of previous pregnancy
History of miscarriage, still birth
History of hemolytic disease of the newborn
Type ABO and Rh and hold
Type and crossmatch
Type and antibody screen
Direct Coombs test
Patient's autologous blood donor
Patient's arranged designated blood donor
Type of blood component requirement
Packed RBC, FFP, PC, cryoprecipitate
Number of cell unit requested
Date and time of requirement
Details of last hemoglobin and PCV value
Diagnosis

13.1.1 Emergency Request

Responsibility for release of emergency assumed by name and signature of the doctor
Release of emergency O group red cells
Patient sample not required
Number and type of cell unit requested

Signature of resident doctor
Name of the doctor
Time and date
Mobile number

P. S. Ajmani, *Immunohematology and Blood banking*, https://doi.org/10.1007/978-981-15-8435-0_13

Approximate time requirement for preparing for a blood transfusion

SN	Procedures	Time
1	Collection of blood from donor	10 min
2	ABO and Rh (D) grouping	10 min
3	Antibody screening	45 min
4	Antibody screening + crossmatching	60 min
5	Antibody identification additional	60 min–24 h
6	Thawing of FFP	20 min
7	Thawing of cryoprecipitate	45 min
8	Washing of erythrocytes	60 min
9	Thawing + washing of frozen RED cells	60 min

The patient's name and medical record number must match with the specimen label. The patient must be positively identified before collection of the blood sample. Check the identification band, and ask the patient to state his/her name and birth date, i.e., "What is your name and birth date?" If the patient is unable to respond, rely on the arm band identification (Tables 13.1, 13.2 and Box 13.1).

13.1.2 Physician Identification

Include the physician's name, ID code number, and mobile number.

Identity of phlebotomist and verifier: with name and signature on blood collection tube and on transfusion requisition form.

13.1.3 Specimen Collection and Labeling of the Tube

At the bedside, before phlebotomy, label the tube with the following pieces of identification. Specimens must be accompanied with a specimen transmittal or clinic encounter form that must match the specimen label. All handwritten requisitions accompanying specimens must have the following legible information (Box 13.2).

Table 13.2 Blood bag receiver slip

Date	Time	Blood bag number	Receiver name and signature
.			

Box 13.1: Identification of the Patient

Blood bank requisition form for patient should have the following information:

First, last, and middle name of patient
Medical record number
Date of birth
Photo ID number
Gender
Address
Date
ICD 10 code: diagnostic information, which establishes medical necessity

Box 13.2: Specimen Collection and Labeling of the Tube

Patient: Last, first, and middle name
Patient medical record number with check digits (eight digits)
Patient's date of birth
Patient residence
Sample collection date and time
Specimen type and/or source
Test required (note any special handling required)
Ordering physician's last and first name

Table 13.1 Blood delivery slip

Requisition received at (time and date)								
Name of the patient		Blood group		Rh (D) group				
Ward number/nursing home								
Details of the blood arranged/supplied								
SN	BB No	Compo	QT	Group	D&T	Compatible	Sign	Issue no
.								
.								
Name, signature of the blood bank officer, and mobile number								

Failure to properly label the tubes will require that the specimens be redrawn. If the patient requires blood as an emergency and another sample cannot be drawn, an **Emergency Release Form** must be signed for uncrossmatched group O blood.

13.1.3.1 Cord Blood Specimens

Requisitions must have both the mother's and the newborn's addressograph imprinted and hospital number. The specimen collected should be clearly identified as cord blood.

Blood testing consists of determining the ABO group and Rh type and performing a direct antiglobulin test (DAT).

Cord bloods are refrigerated and stored for approximately 1 month in blood bank.

13.2 Expiration of the Compatibility Blood Specimen

The expiration of a compatibility specimen only applies to **packed red blood cells (pRBCs).**

For adults, the specimen expires 3 days after the specimen was collected. For example, if the sample was collected on Monday at 2 PM, it would expire Thursday at 2 PM.

For infants, the specimen for infants <4 months expires when the infant turns 4 months of age.

For infant's ≥4 months of age, the expiration of the compatibility specimen follows the same principle as adults.

Blood issued in syringes for pediatric patient expires 4 h after aliquot into the syringe, regardless of the type of component (Boxes 13.3 and 13.4).

Box 13.3: Causes for Specimen Rejection

No label on the tube
Inadequately labeled specimens
Incorrect or incomplete patient identification
Incorrect or incomplete collection of information
Sample collected in wrong tube
Gross hemolysis of blood sample
Diluted or contaminated blood sample received

Box 13.4: Advantages of Uniform Policy for Specimen Acceptance and Rejection

Has a positive impact on patient care
Protects specimen quality
Eliminates risk of exposure to the healthcare worker
Complies with all accreditation standards

13.3 Transport of Blood

Routine: Blood samples may be transported to the blood bank via the messenger service mobile number.

Blood samples may be sent through the pneumatic tube system (tube station).

Emergency—Designate a paramedical individual to carry the patient's sample to the blood bank and return with the blood product(s).

13.3.1 Emergency Requests

Sign under "Responsibility Assumed By _______." Call blood bank in charge to release blood before completion of crossmatch. The signature of the ordering physician is mandatory.

13.3.2 Test Requests

Fill in diagnosis and indicate test requested.

Transfusion Requests: Fill the blood bank requisition form.

13.3.3 Test Results and Product Availability

Results of pretransfusion testing and administration of blood, diagnostic studies, and all patient medical record should be available in the LCR ("Lifetime Clinical Record").

The "Lifetime Clinical Record" is maintained by the Hospital Information Systems (HIS).

A **Lifetime Clinical Record (LCR)** is a component of a digital **electronic health record**

(EHR) system that is used to support modern **medical** care and evaluation. It represents a **clinical** database or a centralized data warehouse for patient **records**.

Authorized number of blood units or blood bank process, i.e., type and antibody Screen (T&S), is expected to be sufficient for at least 90% of the specified elective surgical procedures.

13.4 Request for Delivery of Blood: Ordering

Telephone the blood bank in charge and provide the following information:

- Patient's first and last name or trauma name/number
- Hospital medical record number
- Ward or clinic
- Your name (who has ordered for supply of blood)

13.4.1 Transport of Blood

Routine: When the consultant in charge of the case orders blood products, the blood bank will arrange for delivery via the Messenger Service on mobile SMS. On receipt of the blood, consultant/resident of the case should sign the messenger delivery form with date and time.

Emergency: In emergencies, the responsible physician should designate a paramedical person to transport the blood specimen to the blood bank, wait for uncross-matched blood to be issued, and return with the units to the patient.

Anyone who comes to pick up ordered blood products from the blood bank window must identify in writing the name and medical record number of the patient for whom the blood product(s) is (are) intended. This safety check will be enforced at all times and under all circumstances, including emergency requests and massive transfusion.

Returning unused blood: If blood is not transfused, it must be returned to the blood bank within 30 min of the time that it was issued.

Blood must be stored in a blood bank-monitored refrigerator with an alarm. The only refrigerator outside the blood bank that is suitable for blood storage is located in the operating room area. Unit refrigerators are not suitable for blood storage.

13.5 Administration of O Group Blood Policy

Transfusion of ABO compatible versus ABO identical red cell products:

Group O packed red cells should only be used for group A, B, or AB recipients, if:

- ABO group specific blood is not available.
- Recipient specimen is not available.
- Patient is a neonate.
- Before changing from group O to group specific blood, **the infusion set must** be changed.
- Rh-negative blood may be administered to Rh-positive patients.

13.6 Blood Issuing Policy Protocols

13.6.1 Order of Blood Unit Issuance

When available, the blood bank should issue the blood units in the following order for each patient (in each category, the oldest units will be issued first):

- Autologous unit
- Designated unit
- Regular volunteer unit

Testing protocol: Specimens from patients who are scheduled for elective surgery the following day must reach the blood bank by 10 AM on the day preceding surgery.

Antibody screen positive: If an antibody is detected, blood may not be available at the time requested.

Maximum surgical blood order schedule (MSBOS): Requests received by blood bank that

Box 13.5: Name of the Blood Products Available Through the Blood Bank

Packed red blood cells
Fresh whole blood
Apheresis platelets (AP)
Fresh frozen plasma (FFP)
Thawed fresh frozen plasma
Cryoprecipitate

are not in accordance with the MSBOS list (maximum authorized units of blood available for elective surgery).

Washed red cell units or apheresis platelet units and CMV seronegative are not always available, and their demand should reach the blood bank as per hospital policy.

Other considerations: If it is anticipated that the transfusion will exceed 4 h, special arrangements should be made with the blood bank to split the unit prior to transfusing.

CMV-negative red blood cells will be supplied for infants less than 4 months of age (Box 13.5).

13.6.2 Common Blood Bank Orders

Packed RBC need is unknown: Specimen should be held for 3 days "just in case." No testing is done unless requested.

Type and screen: RBC need is possible. Specimen should be typed for ABO-Rh grouping and screened for RBC antibodies. Type and antibody screen (T&S) is expected to be sufficient for at least 90% of the specified elective surgical procedures.

Type and crossmatch: Means RBC need is likely or definite. T&S should be performed, and request for RBC crossmatched should be reserved.

13.6.3 Turnaround Times for Supply of Blood

Routine: Type and screen for ABO and Rh, 15 min.

Antibody screen: 60 min.

Crossmatch: 30 min.

STAT: Uncrossmatched O-negative, packed RBCs, 5 min.

Uncross-matched type: specific RBCs, 5 min.

Directed transfusion is the collection of blood from donor relative known to the patient and supply of the donor blood to patient if it is crossmatched. In this case donor identity is known by the recipient. Confidentiality has been surrendered in this system.

Advantages: Positive psychological benefit to the patients and donor.

It will increase the blood supply by stimulating more first-time donors and to eliminate fear of blood donation. Once donated, the donor can be recalled to make future blood donations.

13.6.4 Other Important Information

All components issued shall be returned if not transfused so that the patient's transfusion record in the blood bank can be modified to accurately reflect the products given and to avoid unnecessary charges to the patient. Any unit issued is considered transfused, and the patient is charged unless the product is returned to the blood bank.

13.7 Specimen Requirements

Laboratory test results are dependent on the quality of the specimen submitted.

- **Pearl white-top tube plasma preparation tube (PPT)**
- This tube contains EDTA and a special polyester material—used for the collection of plasma for molecular (PCR) tests.
- **Yellow-top tube (ACD)**
- This tube contains ACD, used for the collection of whole blood for special test.
- **Lavender-top tube (EDTA)**
- This tube contains EDTA as an anticoagulant—used for most hematological and blood banking procedures. These tubes are preferred for molecular tests. Tubes with various draw

volumes are available (2.0, 3.0, 5.0, and 0.75 mL microvettes).

- **Red-top tube, glass**
- This tube is a plain glass vacutainer containing no clot activators, anticoagulants, preservatives, or separator material. These tubes can be used for blood bank test.

13.7.1 Blood Specimen Collection and Processing

The first step in acquiring a quality lab test result for any patient is the specimen collection procedure. The venipuncture procedure is complex, requiring both knowledge and skill to perform. Several essential steps are required for every successful collection procedure:

13.7.1.1 Venipuncture Procedure

A phlebotomist must have a professional, courteous, and understanding manner in all contact with all patients.

The first step to the collection is to positively identify the patient by two forms of identification; ask the patient to state and spell his/her name and birth date. Check these against the requisition (paper or electronic).

Check the requisition form for requested tests, other patient information, and any special draw requirements. Gather the tubes intended for the test advised.

Position the patient in a chair or sitting or lying on a bed.

Wash your hands.

Select a suitable site for venipuncture, by placing the tourniquet 3–4 in. above the selected puncture site on the patient.

Do not put the tourniquet on too tightly, or leave it on the patient longer than 1 min.

Next, put on non-latex gloves, and palpate for a vein.

After selection of the vein, cleanse the area in a circular motion, beginning at the site and working outward. Allow the area to air dry. After the area is cleansed, it should not be touched or palpated again. If you find it necessary to reevaluate the site by palpation, the area needs to be re-cleansed before the venipuncture is performed.

Ask the patient to make a fist; avoid "pumping the fist." Grasp the patient's arm firmly using your thumb to draw the skin taut, and anchor the vein. Swiftly insert the needle through the skin into the lumen of the vein. The needle should form a 15–30° angle with the arm surface. Avoid excess probing.

When the last tube is filling, remove the tourniquet.

Remove the needle from the patient's arm using a swift backward motion.

Place gauze immediately on the puncture site. Apply and hold adequate pressure to avoid formation of a hematoma. After holding pressure for 1–2 min, tape a fresh piece of gauze or Band-Aid to the puncture site.

Dispose of contaminated materials/supplies in designated containers.

13.7.1.2 Blood Sample Collection

Collect sample in a screw cap sterile vial with the help of blood bank medical or technical staff on duty.

Label source, sample number, date, and blood group of the donor on sample vial.

Note down sample details in the notebook.

Crosscheck sample details marked on vials with those recorded in notebook. Tighten vial screw cap and keep in refrigerator (at 2–8 °C).

Confirm TTI testing results for collected samples.

Destroy and discard the used gloves.

Biosafety aspects: All blood samples should be considered potentially infectious; hence all biosafety precautions should be followed.

Discard all washing supernatant into 1% sodium hypochlorite.

Ensure that used tips and vials are properly soaked in 1% sodium hypochlorite.

Confirm results for TTIs, and document in register (blood sample collection) and discard as per SOP if found reactive for any TTI.

13.7.1.3 Sample Storage and Documentation

Label blood sample number on respective sample vials and store in refrigerator.

Document sample details in sample collection register.

Confirm test result for collected samples from source as soon as possible, and record in respective register.

Disinfect and discard the sample if vial is broken; reactive for HCV, HIV, HBV, and VDRL; hemolyzed and clotted; and period from date of collection exceeds 35 days.

13.8 Pretransfusion Check: To Be Checked at the Bedside

13.8.1 Procedure

Once all information is checked and found to be correct, resident doctor or BBO should sign the crossmatch transfusion tag.

Identification of the patient and blood product should be confirmed at each stage of the transfusion process by the resident doctor or nurse depending on the hospital policy.

Check the identity of the patient by arm band, Aadhaar card, or voter ID card or any other document.

Check the patient's identification, and ask the patient to state his/her name and birth date (if responsive). These must match exactly the information on the patient's wristband and any other associated paperwork required at the stage of the blood transfusion process.

For patients who are unable to respond entirely or are unconscious or confused, verification of the patient's identification should be obtained from a parent or carer if present.

In an emergency situation, the patient identifiers may be unknown: In this situation, at least one unique identifier—for example, an emergency number or patient's gender—must be used, or follow hospital policy.

If there are patient identification discrepancies at any stage of the transfusion process, the information must be verified, and discrepancies investigated and corrected before proceeding to the next stage of the process.

Compare the ABO, Rh type, and donor number on the blood container label for identical information on the unit tag.

Check the expiration date of the blood.

Check for special requirements where applicable (i.e., leukoreduced, irradiated, CMV negative).

Verify unit as autologous or designated donor by the presence of an extra tag attached to the unit. Autologous is identified by a bright green tag, and the designated donor is identified by a bright orange tag.

Explain to the patient what the transfusion procedure involves.

Inquire as to whether the patient has experienced adverse effects from previous transfusions.

Explain the "transfusion reaction" symptoms to watch, for that should prompt the patient to call for assistance.

Unit is ready for transfusion.

Do not begin the transfusion until all discrepancies have been resolved.

The checker (resident doctor or nurse) must sign his/her name on the first line of the requisition under "Identification Check."

The transfusionist (resident doctor or nurse) must sign his/her name on the second line of the requisition under "Transfusionist."

The signed form must be placed in the patient's chart.

13.9 Ten Golden Rules for Transfusion

- Transfusion should only be used when the benefits outweigh the risks and there are no appropriate alternatives.
- Results of laboratory tests are not the sole criteria for transfusion therapy.

- Transfusion decisions should be based on clinical assessment and supported by laboratory tests.
- Not all anemic patients need transfusion (there is no universal "transfusion trigger").
- Discuss the risks, benefits, and alternatives to transfusion with the patient and attendants and gain consent from any of them.
- The reason for transfusion should be documented in the patient's clinical record.
- Timely provision of blood component support in major hemorrhage can improve outcome—good communication and teamwork are essential.
- Patient's identity must be checked by an ID band (or equivalent) with name, date of birth, and unique ID number.
- The patient must be monitored during the transfusion.
- Education and training underpin safe transfusion practice.

Hemapheresis is defined as collection of whole blood and its separation into different components like platelets, granulocytes, and plasma which are retained and unused blood is returned to the donor.

Therapeutic hemapheresis is the removal of pathological elements or cellular or plasma factors from the blood.

Neonatal hematotherapy: Neonate constitutes first 120 days of life. Sick neonates are subjected to multiple blood laboratory tests which can lead to iatrogenic anemia. In a 1 kg premature, infant may require multiple small volumes 10–15 mL of packed red cell concentrate/kg of body weight. Newborns do not adjust to compensate as rapidly as adults when subjected to hypovolemia or hypoxia.

13.10 Guidelines for the Administration of Blood Products

Inspect the pRBC for presence of clots, unusual discoloration or turbidity, and crack; if found do not use the component unit.

Mix components thoroughly by inversion.

A standard blood giving set incorporating a filter (170–200 μm) should be used for all blood components; these filters remove large clots and aggregates and ensure an effective transfusion flow rate.

Change blood administration set every 12 h if continuing to transfuse or with new IV fluids, or with platelet transfusion, or on completion of transfusion, whichever comes first. One blood administration set may be used for multiple packs of red cells provided flow rate remains adequate and manufacturer's recommendations are not exceeded.

Platelets must be transfused through a new blood administration set. In the setting of massive and rapid transfusion when platelets and plasma are both required, they may be transfused sequentially through the same IV administration set.

Platelets must not be transfused through a blood administration set which has been used for red cells, as red cell debris in the inline filter may trap infused platelets.

Red cells may follow platelets through the same blood administration set, but not precede platelets.

Microaggregate filters (pore size 20–40 μm) are intended to remove microscopic debris from stored red blood cells.

Do not prime, add, or infuse medications or solutions through the same tubing with blood components, except 0.9% sodium chloride injection.

Electrolyte solutions containing calcium, such as Haemaccel®, Hartmann's solution, and lactated Ringer's solution, must never be added to or administered through the same intravenous line as blood components containing citrated anticoagulant. Priming of 0.9% sodium chloride (normal saline) may be required to maintain access if the next red cell unit is not readily available.

13.10.1 Infusion

The recommended rate of infusion of 1 unit of red blood cells is 90–120 min. The transfusion must be completed within 4 h (Tables 13.3 and 13.4).

Table 13.3 Guide for administration of blood and blood components in drops per minute

Component	Volume (mL)	½ h	1 h	2 h	3 h	4 h
		Drops per minute				
Whole blood	400	200	100	50	25	12
pRBC	250	120	60	30	15	15
RBC + additive solution	330	160	80	40	20	20
Washed RBCs	180	100	50	25	25	25
Frozen RBCs	180	100	50	25	25	25
FFP	220	120	60	30	30	30
Deglycerolized RBCs	180	100	50	25	25	25
Plasma	220	120	60	30	30	30
Apheresis platelet	300	160	80			
Platelet concentrate	50	25	Should be completed within 30 min			
Cryoprecipitate	15	20	Should be completed within 30 min			
Leukoreduced RBCs	225	120	60	To be completed in 60 min		
Apheresis granulocyte	220	120	60	To be completed in 60 min		

Whole blood contains 350 mL of blood plus 49 mL of additive solution

Table 13.4 Chart for vital parameters check

Time	Temperature	Pulse	Respiration	BP
Beginning				
30 min				
60 min				
90 min				
120 min				
At completion				

Baseline values for pulse, respiration, blood pressure, and temperature must be obtained and recorded in the patient's chart before beginning the transfusion. Infusion of packed red blood cells should be very slow (approximately 10–25 mL) for the first 15 min. The patient should be observed continuously during this time and then every 30 min to check that the transfusion is proceeding uneventfully. Vital signs must be recorded after 30 min and 1 h and at the end of the transfusion (except in emergencies when rapid transfusion does not permit recording of vital signs at these time points) or when transfusion concludes before the 1-h mark—in this case vital signs must still be recorded at the end of the transfusion.

Administer blood through a filter with normal saline; other solutions may cause hemolysis and/or agglutination.

13.10.2 Monitoring and Observation

Closely observe the patient for the first 15 min of each pack as life-threatening reactions may occur even only a small volume (10 mL) of blood is transfused.

Continue to observe patient BP, pulse rate, heart rate, and respiratory rate regularly throughout the transfusion. When a patient is not under continuous visual observation, consider attending the patient for the first 30 min.

The need for more frequent observations will depend on patient's clinical status.

Do not add medications to blood.

In the case of a transfusion reaction, retain the remainder of any implicated blood.

Outcomes of blood transfusion: select the appropriate clinical outcome of the patient.

If the recipient died following the adverse reaction, enter the date of death whether or not the death was transfusion related.

Enter the relationship of the transfusion to death using the imputability criteria for "Other or Unknown."

Reaction details: Date and time reaction occurred.

For acute reactions, use the date and time the symptoms were first observed.

For delayed reactions, use the date of test identifying new antibodies or date patient noticed symptoms.

If the reaction can be diagnosed, but does not match one of the 12 defined adverse reactions listed, select "Other," and specify the reaction.

13.10.3 Documentation and Traceability

Good documentation of transfusions allows easy and accurate review of records when required for:

- Investigating a transfusion-related adverse event.
- Facilitating donor and recipient "look back" exercises.
- Quality improvement audits.
- Management of legal risk.

13.10.4 Documentation Procedure

The resident doctor on advice of consultant doctor should document the transfusion decision rationale on the basis of clinical guidelines.

Detail the outcome of the informed consent process.

Inform the patient of the potential benefits and risks of transfusion in their particular case and their right to receive or refuse it. Record this decision.

The prescription for blood components and fractionated plasma products is the responsibility of treating doctor.

Document the prescription , and specify blood component or fractionated plasma product to be administered, the quantity, the duration of transfusion, and any special requirements.

A permanent record of the transfusion episode should be kept in the medical notes, including the following:

- Date and time transfusion started and completed
- Type of blood component used and number of units transfused
- Batch number of transfused component
- Signature of resident doctor/nurse administering the transfusion
- Signature of resident doctor/nurse confirming the identity of the patient
- The sheets used for the prescription of blood components or fractionated products
- Nursing observations during the transfusion
- Whether or not the transfusion achieved the anticipated benefit
- Management of any adverse event

All records must be held for the required legislated period.

13.11 Blood Transfusion Documentation

Complete documentation is required at every stage of the blood transfusion process and should include the following steps:

Pretransfusion

- Clinical indication for transfusion
- Date of decision
- Complete blood count (CBC)
- Coagulation profile
- Consent from patient
- Blood component to be transfused and volume

Administration

- Date and time component collected
- Date and time transfusion started
- The donation number of component transfused
- Volume administered
- Name of the nurse who has started the infusion
- Observations before and during transfusion

Posttransfusion

- Date and time component completed
- An indication of whether transfusion achieved the desired effect
- Observations before, during, and after transfusion
- Documentation of any reactions that occurred

Traceability

- All blood components should be traceable from the donor to their final destination.

Further Reading

Brecher ME, editor. American Association of Blood Banks technical manual. 14th ed. Bethesda, MD: AABB Press; 2002.

British Committee for Standards in Haematology, (BCSH) Blood Transfusion Task Force. The administration of blood and blood components and the management of transfused patients. Transfus Med. 1999;9:227–38.

British Committee for Standards in Haematology, (BCSH) Blood Transfusion Task Force. Guidelines for blood bank computing. Transfus Med. 2000;10:307–14.

McClelland DBL, editor. Handbook of transfusion medicine. 3rd ed. London: The Stationery Office; 2001.

Mollison PL. Blood transfusion in clinical medicine. 5th ed. Boston, MA: Blackwell Scientific; 1972.

Petz LD, Swisher SN, Kleinman S, Spence RK, Strauss RG. Clinical practice of transfusion medicine. 3rd ed. New York: Churchill Livingstone; 1996.

Voak D, Chapman JF, Phillips P. Quality of transfusion practice beyond the blood transfusion laboratory is essential to prevent ABO-incompatible death. Transfus Med. 2000;10:95–6.

Walker RH. Special report: transfusion Risks. Am J Clin Pathol. 1987;88:374–8.

14 Blood Bank Inventory

Blood inventory management is an essential part of quality assurance and balance between blood availability and minimizing wastage. The challenge is to keep enough stock to ensure a 100% availability of blood while keeping time expiry losses at a minimum. Optimal management of blood inventory depends on the policies and procedures of blood collection, data collection systems, and effective communication between clinician and blood bank personnel. To operate effectively in the face of both random supply and random demand, sizable buffer stocks of blood and blood components are maintained. The resulting inventory control problem is a complex one for several reasons:

1. Blood is a perishable product. It cannot be stored and used after expiry date.
2. Both supply and demand are random.
3. Voluntary nature and unpredictability of the supply and non-profit nature of the sector.
4. Approximately 30% of all blood demands, "crossmatched" and held for a particular patient, are eventually found not to be required for that patient.
5. Component preparation of blood takes time and is difficult to provide at a short notice.
6. Platelet demands are always increasing, and platelets have short expiry of 5 days and are contaminated easily.
7. Every blood bank interacts with multiple blood bank and hospitals for use of proper blood with short expiry.
8. Increased blood supply demand in cases of natural calamities.

14.1 Wastage

Wastage of blood & its components which is discarded rather than administered to a patient. Ideally it should not be more than 1%.

Types of wastage: It is of two types:

- Firstly there is wastage due to wrongly processed units of blood or test results that indicate that the unit is not safe to use.
- Secondly there is wastage that stems from disposed units that were not used before outdating.

Certain level of blood product wastage is acceptable to ensure products are available when required for patients. Blood bank should monitor

P. S. Ajmani, *Immunohematology and Blood banking*, https://doi.org/10.1007/978-981-15-8435-0_14

and record the wastage of blood products (both expired and discarded products).

14.2 Management

Data analysis of wastage may identify aspects of inventory management which could be improved. For example, high expiry rates may indicate excess blood product stocks are being held or high discard rates may indicate excess blood product stocks are being held or high discard rates may indicate inappropriate practices within hospital wards which may need to be investigated.

Quarantine: The number of certain units of blood components when fully tested and found to be compatible for release to a patient must be kept quarantined or reserved for a specific patient. It should be kept separate from other products that have already been through the testing process and made available.

Quarantine refers to that separation, and it can be both physical (storage in separate portions of a laboratory) and virtual (**Blood Establishment Computer System** or "**BECS**" does not allow a label to be issued for the product until all checks and tests are complete and acceptable).

Blood transfusion service (BTS) should ensure that separate blood storage equipment is clearly designated for:

Unscreened units
Reactive or positive units
Unresolved or undetermined blood component units
Units suitable for clinical use: available blood component stock type and number

Quarantine is also used when a previously acceptable product becomes unsuitable for use or delivery due to a variety of factors, including new post-donation information about the donor of the unit, a test result on a subsequent unit, unusual appearance of blood components or plasma-derived products, or an identified problem with the product (e.g., out of temperature range during transport; positive direct antiglobulin testing (DAT), etc.). The principle is the same: keep the product separate so that it can't be issued in error.

14.2.1 Reasons for Blood Service-Initiated Quarantine

A donor recall, initiated when a donor reports an illness after the donation or when a patient who has received product from the same donor has had a reaction or infection.

14.2.2 Non-conforming Products

The issue of unscreened, partially screened, or non-conforming blood component will only be considered in circumstances where the potential harm of not being transfused is significantly outweighed by the potential risk. The decision for such use ultimately lies with the treating doctor.

14.3 Managing Products with Short Expiry Dates

Platelets have very short shelf lives for 5 days only.

Review component stock and ensure products with a short expiry are used first.

Platelets, which are already allocated to a patient, bring back pre-allocated units with a longer expiry and instead issue units with a short expiry. In case the available stock cannot be used, it can be supplied to other needy blood bank or institution.

First in first out (FIFO) policy: where the oldest blood units are released first.

Last in first out (LIFO): applicable in using an age threshold of 14 days. This requires sufficiency in blood supply.

14.4 Emergency Release of Blood Without Crossmatching

This is a clinical decision determined by the level of urgency and whether the immediate correction of blood loss or anemia outweighs the potential risk of acute or delayed immune hemolysis due to potentially incompatible blood. It is important that a specimen is collected for subsequent pretransfusion testing before blood products are administered.

Emergency release of O Rh-negative blood without sample: Trauma patients with massive hemorrhage will require blood within 5 min of admission to a hospital. It can be supplied without specimen.

14.5 Maximum Surgical Blood Order Schedules (MSBOS)

The available shelf life of a unit of blood component decreases each time the unit is reserved or crossmatched for a patient who does not subsequently receive it. When more blood is crossmatched and set aside for a patient than is required, it is unavailable for other patients and increases the chance that the blood will expire before being used.

The MSBOS identifies the number of units typically required by 80–90% of the patients undergoing a specific surgical procedure where transfusion is likely. This assists the clinician in ordering the appropriate number of units of blood for their patient (Tables 14.1 and 14.2).

Table 14.1 Monthly denominator reporting form

Blood components	No of units issued
pRBCs	
Fresh frozen plasma	
pRBCs without buffy coat	
pRBCs leukocyte depleted	
Random donor platelet	
Pooled platelet unit	
Apheresis platelet	
Cryoprecipitate	
Solvent detergent plasma	
Hospital code Month/year	

14.5.1 Daily Inventory of Blood Stock in Quarantine

- Previous day opening stock + previous day collections from voluntary donors + replacement donors + blood units received from other branches = total available blood stock
- Previous day collections stock − issues to hospitals − expired date stock + non-serological discards, serological discards (HIV, Hep B), or other = new available stock stock = closing stock in quarantine carried forward

14.5.2 Documentation of Inventory Traceability and the Blood Service

Hospital blood bank should maintain transfusion and inventory of products received and their fate so that the final outcome of all components and products is known.

14.6 Importance of Data Collection

Data are an essential tool for evaluation of performance and for developing strategies for improvements and for future planning and for effectively managing the blood inventory management system. A system needs to be developed for the easy retrieval of data associated with transfused patients. It can identify area of growth and problem. Data can help in ensuring blood components are available in a timely manner, in performance benchmarking against its peers, and in monitoring

Table 14.2 Chart showing availability of stock

Analysis of stock							
Group	Rh positive		Rh negative				Total
	WB	pRBC	WB	pRBC	FFP	Platelet	
O							
A							
B							
AB							
Date:	Time:	Signature of BBO					

Box 14.1: Data Collected Should Include

Product
Unique or batch number
Blood group
Expiry date
Date received
Fate of item transfused with patient's name
Date

safety requirements. To enable effective blood inventory management, appropriate data need to be collected across the whole supply chain including voluntary donor and blood donation camps, hospitals, clinician's prescribers, and recipient patients. Collecting and using appropriate data from each of the area can lead to better understanding of the elements of the supply chain and ultimately to improvements in inventory management service. The benefits of data collection far outweigh any problems that might be associated with their collection (Box 14.1).

Supply chain management (SCM) can be defined as the system that effectively plans and manages all activities involved with sourcing and procurement of blood, blood components, supply to hospitals, patients, and all logistics management activities within and between blood bank and pharma company.

14.7 Data from Supply Chain Area from Blood Collection Information from the Donor

Number of blood supply from voluntary donors
Number of blood supply from replacement donors
Number of donors attending the blood bank
Total number of donor bleed
Number of donor not bleed
Number of donor's refuge for donation
Future trend for availability of donors

14.8 Data from Blood Processing and Issue Information

Blood losses due to processing errors
Number & type of outdated units of whole blood & its components
Number and type of units issued to hospital
Number of order not met
Shelf life of blood component stocks

14.9 Data from Hospital Inventory Management

To monitor the inventory level and identify the reasons for potential shortfalls.

To identify the number of wastages due to expiry of components.

Steps taken to rectify the problem area.

Number of transfusion performed.

To analyze the **Issuable Stock Index (ISI)** (day's worth of stock) and wastage in relation to data continuously collected by **blood stock management scheme** (BSMS). The BSMS collects blood inventory data from blood bank and treating hospital.

14.9.1 Measures

The Issuable Stock Index (ISI) is an approximation of the number of days of unreserved stock of all blood groups held in the inventory—**and wastage as a percentage of issues (WAPI)** should be used to present stock and wastage data (hospitals and blood services) in a comparable format. They can also be used as indicators of a hospital inventory management performance.

It is the responsibility of blood bank officer to ensure that donated blood is used efficiently and effectively and to minimize waste while always having sufficient stock available to deal with unexpected life-threatening emergencies. Achieving these goals can be very difficult.

Outdating of component stock is found to be the largest cause, and decrease in discarding rate will be observed after adoption of strategies.

Demand of blood components: To monitor the level of demand for blood and blood components and to identify any shortfall between supply and demand. The insufficient number of donors and increased demand for whole blood and its components are the principle reasons for the short supply. Data collection analysis can help in understanding and addressing some of the reasons for short supply.

The number and reasons for transfusion: To monitor the number of transfusions and identify the reason for transfusion.

Feedback: It is important because of increased participation and it will identify actions that need to be taken.

Management of blood collection: Whole blood collection targets are set annually in advance for anticipated needs and planning purposes. Target needs to be flexible to manage any increase in demand and/or donor attendance shortfalls or over-collection. The collected data is used for target setting and monitoring the supply and the inventory.

Approaches to demand forecasting: Past and current usage of data is crucial for demand forecasting. Long-term demand (4+ years) is difficult to forecast accurately because of voluntary nature of supply. Short-term (up to 2 years) demand forecasts can be made using mathematical modelling techniques. Demand beyond 70 days (2 × 35-day shelf life) is unpredictable.

Contingency and disaster planning: Blood inventory data from hospitals is the key factor in the development of inventory reduction and holding recommendations associated with an integrated blood shortage plan. Hospitals that have taken action on appropriate usage will contribute less in a shortage, and therefore data on wastage and group O usage will be used for benchmarking purposes.

Daily hospital component requirement: Stock data of all the blood components submitted to the BSMS is used to establish the normal daily use of each blood group by an individual hospital in the event of a shortage. The figure is recalculated on a monthly basis and issued by email.

Group	Packed RBC	FFP	Platelet	Platelet concentrate
Availability				
O positive	30	27	25	4
O negative	05			
B positive	20			
B negative	3			
A positive	16			
A negative	02			
AB positive	03			
AB negative	01			

Hospital weekly variation against present inventory: The data show daily hospital usage for all blood groups and their variance against the recommended use. In the event of a shortage, the data will be used to monitor hospital red cell usage.

14.10 Integrated Blood Shortage Plan Benchmarking

Red cell wastage and group O usage data will be used to benchmark hospitals to ensure a fair allocation of blood in the event of a shortage (Box 14.2).

Box 14.2

Country	Annual growth	5-year growth	10-year growth

Issuable stock index wastage as a % of issue:

Further Reading

Aandahl GS, Knutsen TR, Nafstad K. Implementation of ISBT 128, a quality system, a standardized bar code labeling of blood products worldwide, electronic transfusion pathway: four years of experience in Norway. Transfusion. 2007;47(9):1674–8.

Australian and New Zealand Society of Blood Transfusion Ltd and Royal College of Nursing Australia. Guidelines for the administration of blood products. 2nd ed. Australia: Australian and New Zealand Society of Blood Transfusion Ltd and Royal College of Nursing Australia; 2011. Archived from https://anzsbt.org.au/wp-content/uploads/2018/06/ANZSBT_Guidelines_Administration_Blood_Products_3rdEd_Jan_2018.pdf.

Blood Observational Study Investigators on behalf of the ANZICS-Clinical Trials Group. Transfusion practice and guidelines in Australian and New Zealand intensive care units. Intens Care Med. 2010;36:1138–46.

Brodheim E, Derman C, Prastacos G. On the evaluation of a class of inventory policies for perishable products such as blood. Manag Sci. 1975;21(11):1320–5.

Chapman JF, Hyam C, Hick R. Blood inventory management. Vox Sang. 2004;87:143–5.

Funk DM, Lippi G, Favaloro EJ. Quality standards for sample processing, transportation, and storage in hemostasis testing. Semin Thrombosis Hemostasis. 2012;38(06):576–85.

Jennings JB. An analysis of hospital blood bank whole blood inventory control policies. Transfusion. 1968, 8(6):335–42.

Jennings JB. Blood bank inventory control. Manag Sci. 1973;19(6):637–45.

Katsaliaki K. Cost-effective practices in the blood service sector. Health Policy. 2008;86(2–3):276–87. https://doi.org/10.1016/j.healthpol.2007.11.004.

Stanger SH, Yates N, Wilding R, Cotton S. Blood inventory management: hospital best practice. Transfus Med Rev. 2012;26(2):153–63.

World Health Organization. WHO guidelines on drawing blood: best practices in phlebotomy. World Health Organization; 2010. [17 August 2012]. http://www.who.int/entity/injection_safety/job_aids/en/.

Transfusion Reactions 15

Over a period of time, our understanding on blood groups has evolved to encompass not only transfusion-related problems but also specific disease association with RBC surface antigens.

15.1 Definition of Transfusion Reactions

A transfusion-related adverse reaction is a response or effect in a patient associated with the administration of whole blood or blood components. All transfusion reaction should be reported in the transfusion reaction form to blood bank officer.

15.1.1 Report of Adverse Transfusion Reaction to Blood Bank Officer

If consultant in charge of the case suspects or is sure this reaction is the result of an attribute specific to the donor or the blood product, then he has to complete the transfusion reaction form and forward to blood bank officer of the hospital.

Reporting Information

- Submission date of form
- Name of the doctor who has filled the transfusion reaction form
- Title of the doctor who is in charge of the case
- Mobile number of resident and consultant doctor
- E-mail of resident and consultant doctor

For Blood Bank Officer

- Name of the BBO and mobile number
- Case identification number
- Date of receipt of transfusion reaction form along with donor blood transfusion bag, transfusion set, and patient's sample. Approximately remaining blood product at the time of returning blood bag number

Patient's Information

- Hospital code number
- Medical record number (MRN) number
- Patient's first name Gender Age
- Consultant in charge of the case Mobile number
- Hospital admission number
- Primary diagnosis
- Indication for transfusion

P. S. Ajmani, *Immunohematology and Blood banking*, https://doi.org/10.1007/978-981-15-8435-0_15

- Was the patient under anesthesia during transfusion: Yes/no
- Type of anesthesia: GA/spinal/LA
- Relevant severe comorbidity if applicable
- Pertinent medications given
- List transfusion history within 24 h prior to reaction
- List transfusion history within 24 h after reaction
- Any prior history of transfusion reaction: time and date

Current Status at the Time of Reporting
- Returned to pretransfusion status
- Still required medical treatment related to transfusion reaction
- Expired (transfusion-related fatality)
- Expired not transfusion related (Table 15.1)

Reaction Information
- Date and time of transfusion started
- Date and time of reaction started
- Date and time of transfusion stopped (Tables 15.2, 15.3, 15.4, 15.5 and 15.6) (Boxes 15.1 and 15.2)

Transfusion reactions: Whole blood and each blood component transfused carry a small

Table 15.1 Transfusion product detail information

Name of blood bank				
Component	Unit no	Expiry	Volume transfuged	First time/repeat
Whole blood				
pRBC				
Apheresis platelets				
Platelets pooled				
FFP				
Cryoprecipitate				

Table 15.2 Reactions and vital signs

Parameters	Pretransfusion	During transfusion	Posttransfusion
Date and time			
Temperature			
Systolic BP			
Diastolic BP			
Pulse			
Respiratory rate			
O_2 saturation			

Table 15.3 Patient's signs and symptoms at the time of reaction

Generalized	Urticaria	Hypertension	Anuria
Fever	Itching	Arrhythmias	Cough
Chills	Edema	Impending doom	Dyspnea
Rigors	Chest pain	Raised JVP	Wheeze
Nausea	Abdominal pain	Shock	Hypoxemia
Vomiting	Back pain	Wide PP	Headache
Restlessness	Flank pain	Hematuria	Erythema
Anxiety	Substernal pain	Hemoglobinuria	Hoarseness
Jaundice	Hypotension	Oliguria	Fainting

Table 15.4 Laboratory diagnostics—enter values

	Pretransfusion	Posttransfusion
O_2 sat ≤ 90% on room air		
PaO_2/FiO_2 ≤ 300 mmHg		
Chest X-ray: bilateral infiltrates		
Elevated BNP *(value in pg/mL)*		
Elevated central venous pressure greater than 12 mmHg *(value)*		
Elevated pulmonary artery pressure >18 mmHg *(values)*		
Positive fluid balance *(in mL)*		
Transient decrease of white blood cell count		

Table 15.5 Treatment and clinical course

Medication	Treatment given	Response to treatment
Acetaminophen		
Antihistamines		
Bronchodilators		
Diuretics		
Epinephrine		
Intubation/ventilatory support		
Oxygen supplementation		
Steroids		
Vasopressors		
Others		

Table 15.6 Interpretation of transfusion report by blood bank officer

Reaction	Allergic, anaphylaxis, TRALI, TACO, septic, others
Case definition criteria	Definitive, probable, possible
Severity	Non-severe, severe, life-threating, death
Imputability	Definite, probable, possible, doubtful, rule out
BBO name mobile number and e-mail	

Box 15.1: Suspected Adverse Reaction: Assign Priority If More Than One Possibility

Allergic reaction minor
Allergic reaction moderate
Allergic reaction acute anaphylaxis
TRALI
Septic
Others

Box 15.2: Outcome of Transfusion Reaction

Recovered
Recovered with sequele
Permanently disabled
Death

Box 15.3: Potentially Significant and Life-Threatening Reactions Include

Acute hemolytic transfusion reaction
Delayed hemolytic transfusion reaction
Transfusion-transmitted bacterial infection (TTBI)
Anaphylaxis
Transfusion-related acute lung injury (TRALI)

Box 15.4 Common Causes of Transfusion Reactions

Misidentification of the patient
Improper sample identification
Wrong blood issue
Blood administration error
Technical error
Storage error

risk of an adverse effect. Fever, chills, and urticaria are the most common manifestations of transfusion reactions (Box 15.3).

It is important to recognize, respond to, and report adverse events (Box 15.4).

15.2 Classification and Types of Transfusion Reactions

15.2.1 Immediate Immunological Mechanisms

- Fatal-acute hemolytic reaction (ABO incompatibility) mortality: 3.5%
- Non-fatal acute hemolytic reaction (ABO incompatibility) incidence: 1:33,000
- Febrile non-hemolytic reactions (WBC or cytokine induced): 1:200
- Allergic reactions minor (urticarial): 1:300
- Allergic reactions (fatal): Anaphylaxis rare
- Acute non-cardiogenic pulmonary edema (transfusion-related acute lung injury (TRALI)): 1:5000
- Hemolytic transfusion reaction: 1:200
- Transfusion-related acute gut injury (TRAGI): Rare

15.2.2 Immediate Non-immunological Mechanisms

- Circulatory overload common: 1:100
- Non-immunological hemolysis (heat, cold, osmotic, mechanical): Infrequent
- Reaction to bacterial contamination: Uncommon
- Electrolyte imbalance (K, Mg, Ca): Uncommon
- Chemical effects citrate: Uncommon
- Coagulopathy with massive blood transfusion: Uncommon
- Hypotensive transfusion reaction: Uncommon

15.2.3 Delayed Immunological Mechanisms

- Delayed hemolytic reactions alloimmunization (RBC hemolysis and platelet refractoriness): 1:500
- GvHD: Uncommon
- Posttransfusion purpura: Rare
- Trim: Rare

15.2.4 Delayed Non-immunological Mechanisms

- Alloimmunization RBC hemolysis and platelet refractoriness: 1:500
- Delayed hemolysis: 1:4000 rare
- Transfusional hemosiderosis: Rare

15.2.5 Transfusion-Transmitted Infections

Infections: viruses, bacteria, parasite.

Contaminant: Uncommon.

Isoimmmune major transfusion reactions occur immediately and are due to transfusion of ABO-incompatible blood, and laboratory findings are due to complications of hemolysis, DIC, acute renal failure, and cardiovascular failure.

Alloimmune minor transfusion reactions are due to sensitizations of RBCs against foreign, minor, non-ABO antibodies; they are delayed in nature and occur most often 3–10 days after infusion and produce extravascular hemolysis.

15.3 Acute Hemolytic Transfusion Reaction (AHTR) Also Known as Intravascular Hemolytic Transfusion Reaction (AIVHTR)

It occurs during or within 24 h of cessation of transfusion.

It is the most important complication of blood transfusion.

It occurs most commonly due to ABO and Rh (D) blood group incompatibility.

ABO incompatibility results in more severe reaction compared to Rh incompatibility.

It can also occur due to improperly stored blood or hemolyzed blood.

Incompatibility could be due to destruction of donor red cells and recipient's red cells.

Majority of incompatibility reactions results from destruction of donor cells.

Red cell destruction can be intravascular or extravascular, and this depends on the type of antibody involved.

IgM antibodies activate the complement and hence have lytic properties resulting in intravascular hemolysis, whereas IgG antibodies cause phagocytosis by the cells of reticuloendothelial system resulting in extravascular hemolysis.

Destruction of recipient's cells is less common and classically seen when a sensitized group O blood (containing immune-type IgA and IgG) is transfused to a recipient of another blood group.

The course of hemolytic reaction is characterized by four phases; they are phase of hemolytic shock, post-shock phase, oliguric phase, and diuretic phase.

15.3.1 Phase of Hemolytic Shock

The time of onset of symptoms depends on the rate of hemolysis. As little as 10 mL of blood can cause hemolysis; hence, first 50–100 mL of transfusion should be slow and monitored cautiously. In other instances, symptoms appear after 1–2 h or do not appear at all.

Clinical features depend on the amount and nature of antibodies; antibodies in high titer and ability to bind complement result in severe intravascular hemolysis.

15.3.2 Clinical Presentation

Patient complains of pain in the lumbar region, flushing, throbbing headache, precordial pain, tachycardia, hypotension, breathlessness, nausea, vomiting, and fever with chills. In some cases peripheral circulatory failure can occur.

In 50% of the cases, **hemorrhagic diathesis** develops, which in most cases **is the first manifestation**, resulting in bleeding from venipuncture site and surgical field.

In patients under anesthesia, this reaction is masked; therefore, fall in blood pressure, sharp rise in pulse rate, flushing, sweating, or bleeding should be looked for. Morphine also masks a hemolytic reaction.

Box 15.5: Laboratory Findings

Increased serum bilirubin
Increased serum LDH
Decreased plasma fibrinogen
Decreased haptoglobin
Hemoglobinuria
Hemoglobinemia
Plasma discoloration due to hemolysis
Blood smear reveal spherocyte

15.3.3 Post-shock Phase

Hemoglobinuria and jaundice are the characteristic findings in this stage.

Hemoglobinuria is sometimes transient and present in the first voided urine.

Development of jaundice occurs within 12 h after infusion, and it deepens immediately.

Oliguric phase is characterized by hemodynamic alterations in renal microcirculation leading to stasis, activation of coagulation system, and deposition of fibrin. Acute tubular necrosis may occur in few patients. Oliguria is the first sign; it lasts for about 6–12 days but may persist longer.

Diuretic phase: The end of oliguric phase is marked by spontaneous diuresis, signifying recovery. Urinary output increases by 200–300 mL/day. It can lead to excess loss of potassium, sodium, and water and if left uncorrected can be fatal (Box 15.5).

15.3.4 Other Features Are

Immune mediated: Positive direct antiglobulin test (DAT) for anti-IgG or anti-C3 and positive elution test with alloantibody present on the transfused red blood cells.

Non-immune mediated: Negative DAT, and hemolysis is due to physical cause (e.g., thermal, osmotic, mechanical, chemical).

15.3.5 Treatment

Stop transfusion.

Maintain urine output at a rate of 75–100 mL/h by any one of the two:

1. IV mannitol 12.5–50 g given over 5–15 min
2. IV frusemide 20–40 mg

Alkalinize the urine because biocarbonates are preferentially excreted in the urine.

Advice: urine pH determination.

Prevent hypotension to ensure adequate renal blood flow by Rx dopamine >5 μg/kg will cause renal vasoconstriction.

Maintain IV access with suitable crystalloid and colloid solutions.

Maintain an adequate airway.

15.3.6 Monitoring

Monitor renal status by blood urea nitrogen and serum creatinine.

Monitor coagulation status by PT, PTT, and serum fibrinogen.

Monitor for signs for hemolysis (serum bilirubin and LDH).

Hemoglobin value.

The most characteristic sign of an IVHTR is the occurrence of hemoglobinuria and hemoglobinemia

15.4 Febrile Non-hemolytic Transfusion Reactions (FNHTR)

A febrile non-hemolytic transfusion reaction (FNHTR) is defined as a temperature increase of 1 °C over 37 °C occurring during or within 4 h of cessation of transfusion of blood components. This type of transfusion reaction usually occurs at the end of transfusion rather than at the start. It is characterized by fever with chills and rigors, increased respiratory rate, change in blood pressure, anxiety, and a headache; it is usually an isolated finding.

Incidence: FNHTRs are more common due to multiple transfusions of platelet products in multipara women.

Causes: There are two mechanisms involved in the manifestation of an FNHTR. The first involves the presence of a white cell antibody in the patient's plasma that interacts with the white cells in the blood product. These antibodies may be directed against granulocyte antigens or human leukocyte antigens (HLA). This interaction causes endotoxins to be released, which act on the hypothalamus and stimulate a fever.

The second mechanism involves the generation of leukocyte cytokines during product storage. The production of cytokines usually occurs during storage in warmer temperatures.

Management: Clinically assess the transfused patient for fever, chills, rigors, and headache, and rule out appropriately the following three:

- Acute hemolytic reaction
- Transfusion-associated sepsis
- Transfusion-related acute lung injury (TRALI)

Investigation: Complete blood count and repeat ABO grouping.

This type of febrile reaction does not involve red cell reactivity, and direct antiglobulin test (DAT) is negative.

In patients with **repeated FNHTR**, investigation for HLA antibodies may be useful to find out the cause and consider investigations for transfusion-associated sepsis.

Treatment: Stop transfusion immediately.

Treat fever with an antipyretic; avoid aspirin in thrombocytopenic and pediatric patients.

If the patient has history of reaction with previous blood transfusion, then use leukocyte-depleted blood in subsequent transfusion, if indicated.

After the fever has been settled, recommencement of the transfusion, at a slow rate, is possible if other causes of a fever have been excluded.

Consider and exclude other causes, as fever alone may be the first manifestation of a life-threatening reaction.

15.5 Allergic Reaction

They occur in 1–3% of all transfusion reactions. It is a type of hypersensitivity reaction which occurs within seconds or minutes at the start of the transfusion but occasionally may take several hours to develop.

This reaction can range from one lesion to widespread urticarial lesions. This is commonly the only symptom but may be associated with mild upper respiratory symptoms, nausea, vomiting, abdominal cramps, or diarrhea.

It is more common in multi-transfused and multipara. It is non-hemolytic reaction; it is of two types either local reaction or systematic reaction.

Cause: It is caused by IgE-mediated hypersensitivity to allergens or uncharacterized plasma proteins in the transfused unit and mild in nature.

It occurs in the presence of anti-IgA antibodies in patient's circulation which react with IgA of donor plasma.

In some allergic reactions, no specific etiological mechanism can be defined.

Diagnostic criteria for allergic reaction: Two or more of the following occur during or within 4 h of cessation of transfusion:

- Maculopapular rash
- Pruritus
- Generalized flushing
- Edema of tongue, lips, and uvula
- Conjunctival edema
- Erythema and edema of the periorbital area
- Hypotension
- Localized angioedema
- Respiratory distress; bronchospasm
- Urticaria

Investigation: Generally no investigations are required.

If there is more than simple urticaria, hemolysis should be excluded. Indicate direct antiglobulin test (DAT), complete blood count (CBC), and repeat ABO grouping.

Double immunodiffusion assay can be used as a screening test to detect IgA.

Mast cell tryptase test: Levels will peak 1–2 h after symptoms begin.

Tryptase is an enzyme that is released, along with histamine and other chemicals, from mast cells when they are activated as part of a normal immune response as well as in allergic (hypersensitivity) responses. This test measures the amount of tryptase in the blood.

Management: Stop transfusion immediately and Rx 50 mg diphenhydramine or 10 mg chlorpheniramine, and once the reaction subsides, continue transfusion at a slow rate, and complete within 4 h of commencement.

Prevention: Consider premedication with chlorpheniramine for subsequent transfusion if indicated or washed red cells if the patient has recurrent allergic reactions to transfusion. Patient should be closely monitored for severe reaction.

15.6 Severe Allergic Reactions (Anaphylaxis)

This is a rare complication of transfusion of blood components or plasma derivatives.

The risk is increased by rapid infusion, typically when fresh frozen plasma is used.

Reactions usually begin within a few seconds or minutes after the start of the transfusion.

There is sudden onset of severe hypotension, cough, bronchospasm (respiratory distress and wheezing), laryngospasm, angioedema, urticaria, nausea, abdominal cramps, vomiting, diarrhea, shock, and/or loss of consciousness.

No fever.

The incidence is 1:20,000 to 1:50,000 of transfusions.

Causes: This can be caused by any blood product since most contain traces of IgA.

IgA deficiency in the recipient is a rare cause of very severe anaphylaxis.

The following mechanisms have been implicated in anaphylactic reactions.

- IgA-deficient patients having anti-IgA antibodies.
- Patient antibodies to plasma proteins (such as IgG, albumin, haptoglobin, transferrin, C3, C4, or cytokines).
- Transfusing an allergen to a sensitized patient (e.g., penicillin or nuts consumed by a donor).
- Rarely the transfusion of IgE antibodies (to drugs, food, etc.) from a donor to an allergen present in the recipient.

Differential diagnosis: Rule out acute hemolytic transfusion reaction, TRALI, and TACO depending on the clinical picture.

Investigation: Direct antiglobulin test (DAT), blood count, and repeat ABO grouping.

Check the recipient's pretransfusion sample for IgA deficiency and presence of anti-IgA antibodies.

Treatment: Anaphylaxis is likely to be fatal if it is not managed rapidly and aggressively.

Maintain open airway and intravenous line; support blood pressure.

Administer supplemental oxygen, antihistamines, adrenaline, and corticosteroids as required, may require resuscitation.

Further prevention can be done by:

- Advice: no further transfusion of component causing reaction.
- Consider premedication with steroids and antihistamine, if transfusion is further indicated.
- Transfusion of washed red cells or platelets.
- If patient is IgA deficient with anti-IgA, the use of IgA-deficient or washed blood components is recommended.

15.7 Transfusion-Related Acute Lung Injury (TRALI)

It is an acute (<24 h) respiratory immunological transfusion reaction that manifests with fever with chills, dyspnea and dry cough, tachypnea, tachycardia, hypotension, hypoxemia, and non-cardiogenic bilateral pulmonary edema leading to respiratory failure during or within 6 h of transfusion.

Incidence: 1:10,000 the most common cause of transfusion-associated fatalities.

TRALI has been implicated in transfusion of unfractionated plasma-containing components (red cells, platelets, and plasma).

Causes: HNA antibodies—leukocyte **antibodies** against HLA class I and class II and human neutrophil antigens (**HNA**) are formed from exposure to these antigens by transfusion, pregnancy, or transplant and may be associated with transfusion-related acute lung injury (TRALI) and immune neutropenias, resulting in activation and aggregation in pulmonary capillaries, release of local biologic response modifiers causing capillary leak, and lung injury.

Signs and symptoms: Record and observe time of onset of signs and symptoms.

No signs and symptoms of acute lung injury (ALI) before transfusion.

Onset of acute lung injury within 5 h of end of transfusion and hypoxemia is defined by any of these methods:

- PaO_2/FiO_2 less than or equal to 300 mmHg.
- Oxygen saturation less than 90% on room air.
- Chest X-ray will show bilateral pulmonary infiltrates.
- Lack of clinical evidence of left atrial hypertension (circulatory overload).

TRALI has many clinical features in common with TACO and requires careful clinical and laboratory assessment.

Acute hemolytic reaction or transfusion-associated sepsis may have similar initial clinical findings.

Chest X-ray will show bilateral interstitial infiltrates.

Management: Stop transfusion immediately. TRALI is associated with a high morbidity, and the majority of patients require support to maintain blood pressure and to maintain an open airway. Administer supplemental oxygen. As with ARDS, diuretics or corticosteroids are not helpful. The mortality rate of TRALI is reported as high as 20% in general populations and up to 58% in critically ill patient populations. However, with supportive care, the lung injury is generally transient, with oxygen levels returning to pretransfusion levels within 48–96 h and chest X-ray returning to normal within 96 h. However, some patients are slower to recover and may remain hypoxic with persistent pulmonary infiltrates for several days, although pulmonary function eventually returns to baseline without apparent sequelae.

Any blood donors involved in cases defined as TRALI or suspected TRALI are deferred from whole blood or apheresis platelet donation.

Investigations: HLA testing of donor & patient: Patient's pretransfusion serum and post-transfusion samples: 10 mL serum and 20 mL EDTA or ACD samples should be sent to blood bank for investigation labelled as "TRALI" investigations.

Direct antiglobulin test (DAT), complete blood count, and repeat ABO grouping may be indicated (Table 15.7).

Table 15.7 Distinguishing features between TRALI and TACO

Features	TRALI	TACO
Temperature	Increased	Normal
Blood pressure	Decreased	Increased
Neck veins	No change	Can be distended
Heart auscultation	Crepitations	Crepitations +++ and/or s3
Ejection fraction	Normal or decreased	Decreased
Pulmonary artery pressure	<18 mmHg	>18 mmHg
Pulmonary edema nature	Exudate	Transudate
Diuretic therapy	Deteriorate	Improved
IV therapy	Improve	Deteriorate
WBC count	Transient decreased	No change
Brain natriuretic protein	<200 pg/mL	>1200 pg/mL

15.7.1 How to Reduce Risk of Antibody-Mediated TRALI

Do not collect the blood from donors having HLA or HNA antibodies.

Prepare and transfuge blood products prepared from male donors only.

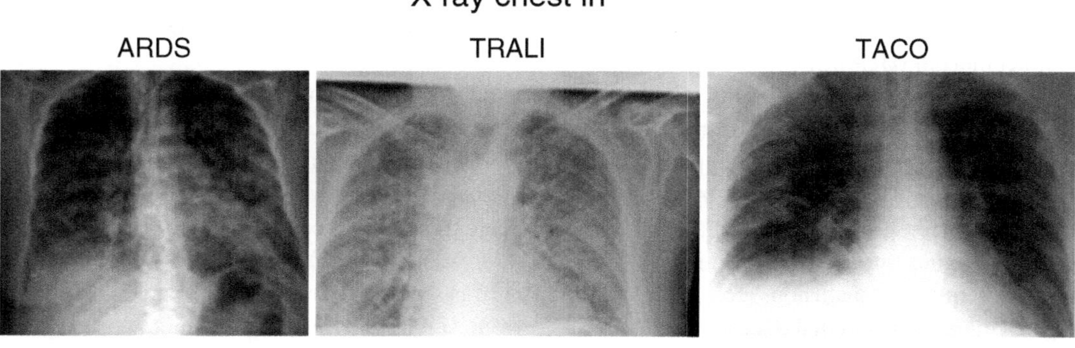

ARDS: Showing bilateral opacities.

TRALI: Showing alveolar and interstitial infiltrates.

TACO: Showing vascular congestion.

15.8 Transfusion-Related Acute Gut Injury (TRAGI)

Transfusion-related acute gut injury is defined as the occurrence of necrotizing enterocolitis within 2 days or less after a packed red blood cell (pRBC) transfusion in old or low-risk infants born at extremely low gestational ages (<28 weeks gestational age).

Transfusion-associated dyspnea (TAD) is an acute respiratory distress occurring within 24 h of cessation of transfusion, and it rules out allergic reaction, TACO, and TRALI definitions.

15.9 Immune-Mediated Chronic Transfusion Reactions

15.9.1 Alloimmunization

It occurs as a result of an immune response after exposure to foreign antigens after blood transfusion, pregnancy, or tissue transplant. This can result in formation of alloantibodies against red cells, human leucocyte antigen (HLA), or human platelet antigen (HPA).

Alloimmunization against red cells results in an acute or delayed hemolytic transfusion reaction and hemolytic disease of the newborn. Approximately 1% of red cell transfusions is associated with alloantibody formation but may be much higher (up to 30%) in patients who frequently required transfusion such as those with sickle cell disease and thalassemia.

HLA and HPA antibody formation may lead to platelet refractoriness leading to insufficient increase in platelet count after infusion of platelet.

It may occur in about 20–70% of patients receiving multiple platelet transfusions. Posttransfusion purpura can also occur as a consequence of development of HPA and HLA antibodies.

Alloimmunization against HLA antigen is also implicated in transplant rejection, febrile non-hemolytic reaction, and TRALI.

Investigation: Obtain patient history of any previous transfusions, transplantations, or pregnancies.

Perform antibody screen tests on the patient's plasma to detect clinically significant red cell antibodies and HLA or HPA antibodies.

Treatment: Treatment depends on the type and severity of the transfusion reaction.

Prevention: Use of leucodepleted blood products.

RhD immunoglobulin is given to pregnant women who are RhD negative to prevent hemolytic disease of the newborn.

To reduce the risk of TRALI, plasma for FFP and cryoprecipitate is only accepted from males and apheresis platelets from males and nulliparous women only.

If a red cell alloantibody is identified, antigen-negative blood is needed in further transfusion.

With patients on long-term transfusion support, such as patients with thalassemia, giving phenotyped matched blood early in their repeated blood support may reduce the risk of further antibody development.

15.9.2 Delayed Hemolytic Transfusion Reaction (DHTR)

It occurs 3 days to 3 weeks (delayed reaction) posttransfusion of a red cell component and is extravascular in nature producing mild clinical picture. The signs and symptoms are similar to an acute transfusion reaction but are less severe.

Incidence: 1:2400 of transfusions.

It is seen more frequently in patients suffering from sickle cell and thalassemia who requires frequent blood transfusions.

15.9.2.1 Causes

After transfusion, transplantation, or pregnancy, a patient may make an antibody to a red cell antigen that they lack. The amount of antibodies in patient's serum is at low level and therefore not detected during pretransfusion screening. If the patient is later exposed to a red cell transfusion which expresses the same antigen, an anamnestic response may occur where the antibody level rises rapidly and hence leads to DHTR.

It is due to sensitization of RBCs against those of the Kidd, Duffy, Kell, and MNS systems, in order of decreasing frequency. The clinical severity of a DHTR depends on the immunogenicity or dose of the antigen.

Clinically the first indication is fever, jaundice, or unexplained fall in hemoglobin.

Diagnosis is confirmed by a positive direct antiglobulin test (DAT) for antibodies developed between 24 h and 28 days after cessation of transfusion **and either** positive elution test with alloantibody present on the transfused red blood cells or newly identified red blood cell alloantibody in recipient's serum **or** inadequate rise of posttransfusion hemoglobin level or rapid fall in hemoglobin back to pretransfusion levels or otherwise unexplained appearance of spherocytes.

15.9.2.2 Investigation

- Direct antiglobulin test (DAT)
- Antibody D titer
- Serum LDH
- Markers of hemolysis: serum haptoglobin, bilirubin

15.9.2.3 Treatment

Most delayed hemolytic reactions have a benign course and require no treatment; however life-threatening hemolysis with severe anemia and renal failure may occur.

Patients suffering from sickle cell disease and thalassemia, who frequently require blood, should have extended red cell phenotyping and receive red cells matched for at least ABO, Rh (D, C, c, E, e), and Kell antigens.

It is important to know that incompatible IV solutions can cause transfusion reactions secondary to cell lysis or agglutination.

15.9.3 Transfusion-Associated Graft-Versus-Host disease (TAGVHD)

It is an extremely rare clinical syndrome occurring from 2 days to 6 weeks after cessation of transfusion characterized by:

- Fever.
- Characteristic rash: erythematous, maculopapular eruption centrally that spreads to extremities and, in severe cases, progresses to generalized erythroderma and hemorrhagic bullous formation.
- Diarrhea.
- Hepatomegaly.
- Increased alanine transaminase.
- Increased aspartate aminotransferase.
- Increased serum bilirubin.
- Increased alkaline phosphatase.
- Bone marrow aplasia.
- Pancytopenia.
- Characteristic histological appearance of skin or liver or bone marrow biopsy is diagnostic.

TA-GVHD leads to pancytopenia of bone marrow with a mortality rate >90%. Death typically occurs within first 3 weeks of first symptoms, most commonly due to overwhelming infections.

15.9.3.1 Causes

It usually occurs in immunodeficient recipients whose immune system is unable to recognize the transfused T lymphocytes as foreign. These lymphocytes engraft in the recipient and react against the host.

Risk factors: Degree of immunodeficiency of the recipient.

Number of viable T lymphocytes transfused (affected by the age of the blood transfused), leucodepletion, and irradiation level of the blood product.

15.9.3.2 Treatment

Treatment is only supported by corticosteroids and cytotoxic drugs, but they are largely ineffective, and therefore, prevention is the treatment of choice.

15.9.4 Transfusion-Related Immune Modulation (TRIM)

It is a transient immunosuppression in recipients which may occur following transfusion of allogeneic blood.

There are no specific signs or symptoms of TRIM and the incidence is unknown.

Causes: The mechanism of immunosuppression is not known. It is partially due to transfused white cells releasing cytokines, which leads to immune modulation.

There have been a number of reported TRIM-associated effects on the transfusion recipient ranging from improved clinical outcome in renal allograft transplantation to an increased rate of tumor recurrence in cancer surgery patients and an increased rate of postoperative bacterial infection.

Investigation: Does not require any specific investigation.

Treatment: No treatment is indicated.

Prevention is to avoid allogeneic blood transfusion. Only transfuge leucodepleted blood products with WBC filter

15.9.5 Posttransfusion Purpura

It is a rare and delayed transfusion reaction which typically occurs 7–10 days after a blood transfusion characterized by sudden onset and self-limiting thrombocytopenia (platelet counts $<10 \times 10^9$/L in 80% of cases) and count returns to normal within 2 weeks

It is five times more common in females who usually have a history of sensitization by either pregnancy or multiple transfusions.

Clinical Presentation: Bleeding from mucous membranes and the gastrointestinal and urinary tracts is common. Mortality is rare but may be due to intracranial hemorrhage.

Causes: It is due to antibodies to platelet-specific antigens, most often **human platelet antigen** 1a (HPA-1a); however antibodies to HPA-1b, other platelet antigens, and **HLA antigens** have also been implicated in PTP.

Investigation: Flow cytometry and fluorescent-labelled polyclonal antibodies specific for IgG and IgM in the patient's plasma are the investigation of choice.

Management: It becomes clinically important at a platelet count of 50×10^9/L, with a danger of hidden (occult) bleeding at 20×10^9/L.

Rx prednisolone 1 g IV.

Rx IV immunoglobulin, 2 g/kg for 1 day or 0.4 g/kg for 5 days.

Patient may require plasma exchange.

Monitor the patient's platelet count: normal range is 150×10^9/L to 440×10^9/L.

If available, give platelet concentrates that are negative for the platelet-specific antigen against which the antibodies are directed.

Unmatched platelet transfusion is generally ineffective.

Recovery of platelet count after 2–4 weeks is usual.

Outcome of the management: The platelet count is expected to rise in the next 4 days. Antigen-negative red cells and platelets may be indicated if subsequent transfusion is required, but this is controversial.

15.10 Non-immune-Mediated Acute Transfusion Reactions

15.10.1 Transfusion-Associated Circulatory Overload (TACO)

It is the second most common cause of death following transfusion, accounting for 21% of all reported fatalities and major morbidity reported. Circulatory overload occurs following infusion of too much blood too quickly leading to pulmonary edema. In normal subject, rapid transfusion in a previously stable patient with normovolemia may cause a transient rise in venous pressure which comes back to normal as soon as it is stopped.

The risk of TACO is higher in elderly, infants, children, and patients with chronic anemia and cardiac and pulmonary disease.

Causes: This is usually due to rapid or massive transfusion of blood in patients with diminished cardiac reserve or chronic anemia.

Incidence: TACO occurs in approximately 1:100 transfused patients.

Diagnosis: New onset or exacerbation of three or more of the following within 6 h (acute onset) of cessation of transfusion:

- Acute respiratory distress (dyspnea, orthopnea, cough).
- Elevated central venous pressure (CVP).
- Elevated brain natriuretic peptide (BNP).
- Evidence of positive fluid balance.
- Evidence of left heart failure.
- Pulmonary edema on chest X-ray.

15.10.1.1 Test for TACO

B-natriuretic peptide (BNP) test: BNP levels are measured using fluorescent immunoassay. It measures levels of a protein BPN that is made by the heart and blood vessels. BNP levels are higher than normal in heart failure. Normal value is BNP 100 pg/mL. BNP value of more than 100 pg/mL has 95% specificity and 98% sensitivity.

Investigation: **TACO** is frequently confused with TRALI. Chest X-ray reveals pulmonary edema in both the cases, but in TACO hypertension is a constant feature, but in TRALI it is infrequent and transient.

Treatment: Stop transfusion immediately, and follow other steps for managing suspected transfusion reactions.

Place the patient in an upright position and treat symptoms with oxygen.

Circulatory overload may require IV diuretics. Monitor the patient's vital signs and urine output carefully.

Oligemia is occasionally seen as engorgement of neck veins and moist sounds on auscultation of chest.

It is prevented by close monitoring of heart rate and blood pressure and also peripheral temperature.

In patients with renal insufficiency: the resulting increase in blood volume is far more prolonged than in normal subjects. Because of this Hb concentration may appear to fail to rise due to the very slow adjustment of blood volume.

In patients with severe anemia: the risk of hypervolemia can be reduced by restricting the rate of transfusion to 1 mL/kg of body weight.

Prevention: In susceptible patients at risk for TACO (pediatric patients, patients with severe anemia, and patients with congestive heart failure), transfusion should be administered slowly, and consideration is given to use of a diuretic.

15.10.2 Non-immune-Mediated Hemolysis

Patients often present with fever and increased pulse rate. The clinical picture varies depending on the amount of component transfused and resulting degree of hemolysis. Most non-immune-mediated hemolysis situations are benign, but life-threatening hemolysis with severe anemia and renal failure may occur.

Hemoglobinuria and hemoglobinemia are common symptoms.

The incidence rate for acute non-immune-mediated hemolysis is rare.

Causes of non-immune-mediated red cell hemolysis include:

- Inadvertent freezing of red cells (transporting directly on ice or storage in freezer).
- Incomplete deglycerolization of frozen red cells.
- Transfusion of red cells under pressure through a small-bore needle.
- Using a rapid pressure infuser.
- Overheating of red cells >30 °C.
- Transfusion of improperly stored blood can lead to DIC and shock.

- Medical device malfunctions (blood warmers or cell savers).
- Improper use of hot water baths to warm blood.
- Infusion of red cells simultaneously through the same tubing with hypotonic solutions, dextrose saline, or pharmacological agents.
- Bacterial contamination of the red cell unit.
- Transfusion of outdated red cells.
- Patient's underlying disease process.

Investigations

- Direct antiglobulin test (DAT) to rule out immune hemolysis.
- Repeat patient ABO grouping.
- Test the transfused unit for hemolysis.
- Identify the root-cause analysis and eliminate the cause.

Platelet transfusion refractoriness (PTR) refers to the repeated failure to achieve satisfactory responses to platelet transfusions from random donors. The cause of refractoriness may be immune <20% or non-immune >80%. Among immune-related refractoriness, antibodies against HLA antigens are the primary cause.

Treatment: One unit (standard adult dose) of apheresis or pooled platelets would be expected to raise the platelet count of a 70 kg adult by 20–40 × 10^9/L.

Continue to transfuse ABO-compatible platelets as required.

PTR is associated with the following adverse outcomes:

- Longer hospital stays
- Increased risk of bleeding
- Higher inpatient hospital costs

15.10.3 Non-immune-Mediated Chronic Transfusion Reactions

Alloimmunization (RBC hemolysis, platelet refractoriness).

Iron overloads (transfusion hemosiderosis): 1 L of blood contains 500 mg iron.

15.10.3.1 Causes

Patients who are chronically dependent on multiple red cell transfusions (e.g., thalassemia, red cell aplasia, aplastic anemia, sideroblastic anemia) will accumulate excess total body iron over time. Excessive iron accumulates and is deposited in parenchymal cells of organs such as the heart, liver, spleen, and endocrine organs and affects their function. Hemosiderosis occurs when more than 100 units of packed red cell concentrate has been administered.

Early symptoms are often vague such as muscle weakness, fatigue, and weight loss. Later skin pigmentation, arthropathy, diabetes, impotence, cardiac failure, and hepatic dysfunction can occur.

Each unit of red cells contains about 250 mg of iron, and the average rate of iron excretion is only about 1 mg/day. Therefore, iron overload can occur after transfusion of about 10–20 units of pRBC units.

15.10.3.2 Investigation

Serum ferritin

MRI which assesses iron concentration in the heart and liver

Liver biopsy

15.10.3.3 Treatment

Treatment is aimed at removal of accumulated iron in the tissues by using iron chelating agents which form a complex with iron and promote its excretion. Rx DFA 500 mg/IM. Desferrioxamine, a chelating agent, lessens the iron overload.

15.10.4 Transfusion-Transmitted Bacterial Infection

Presentation: It usually occurs during the transfusion, and the clinical features suggest the possibility of bacterial contamination and/or endotoxin reaction and shock. It may include rigors, high fever, severe chills, hypotension, tachycardia, nausea and vomiting, dyspnea, or circulatory collapse during or soon after transfusion. In severe cases, the patient may develop shock with accompanying renal failure and disseminated intravascular coagulation (DIC). This reaction may be fatal.

15.10.4.1 Causes

Blood components may be contaminated by bacteria from the donor's skin during the collection procedure, due to improper antiseptic technique.

Undetected bacteremia in the donor.

Contamination from the environment.

Contamination during the preparation of components.

Contamination of platelets occurs more frequently due to its storage temperature at room temperature.

Previously frozen components thawed by immersion in a water bath.

Use of improper stored red cell components.

Both Gram-positive and Gram-negative organisms have been implicated in transfusion-transmitted bacterial infection with serious morbidity and mortality occurring most frequently with Gram-negative bacteria.

Organisms capable of multiplying at low temperatures and those using iron as a nutrient are most often associated with red cell contamination, especially *Yersinia enterocolitica* (Boxes 15.6 and 15.7).

Contamination is suggested by appearances of residue, hemolysis, and rarely a slight smell of hydrogen sulfide when bag is opened.

Box 15.6 Pathogens Causing Bacterial Contamination of Platelets

S. aureus
Klebsiella
Pneumonia
S. marcescens
Staphylococcus epidermidis

Box 15.7 Pathogens Causing Bacterial Contamination of pRBC

Staphylococcus epidermidis
Bacillus cereus
Yersinia enterocolitica

15.10.4.2 Investigation

Culture and Gram stain of the remainder of the blood component. Blood culture of the patient is the key to diagnosing transfusion-related sepsis depends on culturing the same organism from the patient and component.

Keep the blood bag and giving set (sealed) for further investigation. Ensure quarantining and testing of related components from the same donation/donor.

15.10.4.3 Treatment

Stop transfusion immediately.

Start broad-spectrum antibiotics once cultures have been taken.

Patient should be managed by plasma volume expanders, pressor agent, and hydrocortisone.

Death occurs within a matter of hours if not managed.

Provide cardiorespiratory support (Boxes 15.8 and 15.9).

Cytomegalovirus (CMV) causes posttransfusion pyrexia and hepatitis in transplant patients and those on cytotoxic drugs. However, leucode-

Box 15.8: Transfusion-Transmitted Infection (TT)

The list includes five diseases which are screened in every donor to minimize the risk of transmitting infectious agents to patients. They are:

Human immunodeficiency virus (HIV) 1 and 2
Hepatitis C virus (HCV)
Hepatitis B virus (HBV)
HTLV 1 and 2
Treponema pallidum infection

Box 15.9: The following tests are Screened in the Blood Components of Children and Immunocompromised Patients

CMV
Parvovirus B19
EBV

pletion may be equal to CMV seronegativity in the prevention of transfusion transmission of CMV.

Epstein–Barr virus (EBV) commonly causes infectious mononucleosis and may also be transmitted by transfusion.

Occasionally toxoplasma and brucellosis can also be transmitted.

Other viruses which may be transmitted by blood transfusions are dengue virus (dengue fever), West Nile virus, Chikungunya virus, and Parvovirus B19 which causes the "slapped cheek syndrome" or Fifth disease.

Causes: The primary cause of transfusion-transmissible viral infections is thought to be related to donations made by individuals in the window period, which is the interval between the time of infection and the appearance of clinical symptoms or detectable disease markers, such as specific antibodies or viral nucleic acid sequences.

Prevention: While collecting blood from the donors, they should be subjected to stringent screening procedures, including collection of a comprehensive medical and travel history as part of the donor assessment process. For example, the risk of transmitting dengue fever, West Nile, and Chikungunya viruses is minimized by excluding donors from or have recently travelled to areas where the diseases are endemic. Similarly, the risk of transmitting HIV, hepatitis B, and hepatitis C is reduced by excluding donors who engage in high-risk behavior.

However, there are some infectious agents for which routine tests are not readily available to prevent the disease from being transmitted by transfusion. These include Chagas disease and the variant Creutzfeldt–Jakob disease (vCJD) linked to the bovine spongiform encephalopathy (BSE) which is transmitted by a prion.

The residual risk of transmission by transfusion varies according to the incidence of the infection in the donor population and the donor screening processes that are in place.

Clinically assess patients for manifestations of specific viral infections.

Perform appropriate investigations and specific testing for viral markers.

Table 15.8 Risk of hepatitis with different blood components

Highest risk	Average risk	No risk
Factor II	Whole blood	Human albumin
Factor VII	pRBC	Immune globulin
Factor VIII	Single donor platelet	
Factor IX	Plasma	
Factor X		

Following the transfusion of whole blood and blood products, the risk of anicteric hepatitis is much greater than that of clinical hepatitis with jaundice (Table 15.8).

15.11 Transfusion-Transmissible Infection

15.11.1 Malaria

Malaria is a rare transfusion-transmitted infection but continues to pose a risk in developing countries including India.

Presentation: Symptoms may be non-specific such as fever, headache, nausea, vomiting, joint pains, and diarrhea. It should be suspected in any patient with a febrile illness if they had exposure to an area known to be endemic for malaria.

Causes: Malaria is an infectious disease caused by a parasite, *Plasmodium* species. The two common types of plasmodium in India are *P. vivax* and *P. falciparum*. The parasite invades red blood cells and destroys those releasing daughter cells which further invade more red cells. Malaria is transmitted to humans through the bite of the female *Anopheles* mosquitoes. It can also rarely be transmitted through blood transfusion from an infected donor.

Investigation: Suspected malaria is diagnosed by visualization of parasites in blood smears or by detection of parasite antigens or antibodies by rapid diagnostic tests (Box 15.10).

Treatment: Chloroquine is the drug of choice.

Box 15.10 Parasites in Blood

Plasmodium
Babesia
Trypanosoma
Leishmania
Borrelia

15.11.2 Chagas Disease

Chagas disease is a disease transmitted by parasite *Trypanosoma cruzi* and is known to be transmitted by transfusion of fresh blood products. It is endemic in Central and South America, and therefore people born or have received fresh blood products from these areas are restricted to donation of plasma for fractionation only.

Hypotensive transfusion reaction: All other adverse reactions presenting with hypotension are excluded, and hypotension occurs during or within 1 h after cessation of transfusion.

Thrombophlebitis: Infusion failure is defined as failure of an infusion while needed. It is most commonly due to phlebitis and due to extravasation. It is also due to rupture vein wall by the needle tip. It occurs most commonly after cannulation. It is commonly associated with blood transfusion when dextrose or saline is used in addition. The chances of occurring increase when the duration of transfusion is longer. It is seen in patients who live by their veins, like hemophilia and aplastic anemia in whom the cannula is left for a longer time.

Septic phlebitis of cannulated veins may be a grave complication of treatment.

Air embolism: Air can be introduced in the patient's vein during transfusion by failing to expel air. In sick patients 10–40 mL of air can cause alarming symptoms and even death. Strict precautions should be taken to prevent air entry; before commencing a transfusion, air should be driven out of the tubing by running blood through it; a small amount of blood should be left in the pack before changing to the next so that tubing remains full.

Clinically, there is sudden onset of dyspnea, cyanosis, hypotension, weak pulse, and syncope.

Treatment: Patient should be placed on their left side in a head-down position to encourage displacement of air from the right ventricle.

15.12 Non-immunological Reactions

Effect of vaso-active substances: A degradation product of factor XII may cause hypotension, vasodilation, nausea, sweating, and chest pain.

Pyrogens—bacterial and endogenous: They are low molecular weight proteins liberated by leucocytes; stimulation of PGE2 in hypothalamus leads to pyrexia.

Effect of cold blood: Cardiac side effects, ventricular arrhythmias, and extrasystoles have been noted.

Others: If the reaction is not defined in the Hemovigilance Module surveillance protocol (e.g., transfusion-associated acute gut injury (TRAGI), transfusion-associated immunomodulation (TRIM), iron overload, microchimerism, hyperkalemia, thrombosis), it comes under the category of others.

Therapeutic Phlebotomy is the removal of blood from the body, to treat the underlying disease. It is the preferred treatment for blood disorders in which the removal of red blood cells or serum iron is the most efficient method for managing the symptoms and complication such as polycythemia vera, hemochromatosis, and porphyria cutanea tarda.

15.13 Management of Suspected Transfusion Reactions

When possible, before transfusing a patient, the physician should always inquire about a history of previous transfusions, pregnancies, allergies, and possible transfusion reactions.

Stop the transfusion, and check all labels, forms, and patient identification to determine if the patient received the correct blood.

Keep the IV line open with normal saline. If the patient has had previous mild allergic reactions, i.e., localized urticaria without breathing difficulties or hypotension, administer antihistamine chlorpheniramine 0.01 mg/kg IM, or Benadryl may be given IV for symptomatic relief (not to be given through the transfusion line).

If the patient has a mild febrile reaction, additional medication with an antipyretic may control it, and allow continued transfusion after a hemolytic reaction has been ruled out.

Collect urine for the next 24 h for evidence of hemolysis; if patient responds well with clinical improvement, restart transfusion slowly with new RCC unit.

If there is no clinical improvement within 30 min or if signs and symptoms worsen, treat as category II reactions.

Febrile reactions may (very rarely) be caused by bacterial sepsis from contaminated blood products. If it is due to contaminated blood products, stop the transfusion immediately, and send the blood products to blood bank for further investigations.

In reactions where respiratory symptoms dominate, volume overload and TRALI should be considered. The latter may respond to simply stopping or slowing down the transfusion or may require IV diuretics. TRALI often requires ventilatory support. When respiratory distress and circulatory collapse are both present, within seconds to a minute after blood product administration, anaphylaxis should be considered and requires emergency treatment. For possible red cell reactions and/or anaphylactic reactions, monitor vital signs and urine output till patient recovers. Start appropriate fluid and pressor therapy for the rare hemolytic or anaphylactic reactions. Intravenous corticosteroids may be considered to prevent worsening of acute reactions due to hemolysis or anaphylaxis. Heparin may have a role in managing acute DIC. Critical care, renal, hematology, and blood bank physicians should be consulted as appropriate for advice on management of severe cases.

15.13.1 Life-Threating (Category 3) Reactions

Give adrenaline (as 1:1000) solution by intramuscular route.

Administer IV prednisolone and bronchodilators.

Reassess the condition of patient if hypotension persists:

- Continue IV saline.
- Give dopamine IV infusion 1 g/kg/min.

In case of falling urine output:

- Continue frusemide.
- Continue dopamine.
- The patient may need renal dialysis.

15.14 Investigation of Transfusion Reaction

If the patient indicates the signs of hemolytic reaction, stop further transfusion, and it can be life-threatening and should be treated on a STAT basis, and proceed for investigation.

Report all transfusion reactions promptly to blood bank officer on transfusion reaction report form. Document the findings on the patient's chart. The blood bank resident will review the case and prepare a report for the electronic medical record (LCR) (Box 15.11).

15.14.1 Clerical Check

Check all relevant paper work—the number of units transfused, identification of the patient, crossmatching reports, records of previous transfusions; ensure that transfusion was without fault and any clerical error. The most common cause of transfusion reaction is the infusion of wrong blood to the wrong patient and misidentification of the patient.

Box 15.11 Three Basic Preliminary Tests in Blood Bank Laboratory

Cleric check
Visual check
Serology check

Other causes are mix-up of blood samples in the laboratory and blood is supplied without crossmatching.

15.14.2 Visual Check

Immediately upon receipt of clamped blood bag with unused blood and attached blood administration set, inspect for hemolysis, purple discoloration, clot formation, cloudy appearance, clumps of RBCs, and/or any evidence of contamination of blood or blood components. Inspect both blood bag and blood transfusion set separately. If positive then perform Gram stain and culture examination. Culture samples should be taken from the returned blood bag and from the pilot tube.

Collect 10 mL of patient blood from another arm, and send it for culture examination for both Gram-positive and Gram-negative organisms.

Take a swab from the patient infusion arm, and prepare a Gram stain for confirmation of sepsis. Preserve the clamped blood bag with any unused blood, and attach administration set for retesting of ABO-Rh typing or further testing.

Keep the crossmatching tubes (pilot tubes) and patient's sample for at least 7 days following transfusion for further testing.

Collect 10 mL of patient blood after transfusion reaction, and allot it to stand at room temperature. Separate serum and red cells into two different tubes, and label them accordingly. Care should be taken to avoid hemolysis.

Collects the patient's urine 1, 2, and 3 h after transfusion, and examine for hemoglobinuria. Take 10 mL of urine in a glass tube, and centrifuge at 1500 rpm for 5 min. Prepare a smear with the sediment and see the presence of red cells. Perform this procedure with all the three samples. Presence of red cells is indicative of hemoglobinuria. Quantify hemoglobinuria as mild, moderate, and severe indicating the threshold of reaction.

Transfer the blood from the donor set in a small glass test tube, and centrifuge at slow speed, and observe the plasma for any sign of hemolysis of red cells, and compare with the posttransfusion sample of the patient. This step is done to rule out hemolysis. Destruction of red cells will release hemoglobin resulting in pink- or red-colored serum (Boxes 15.12 and 15.13).

Box 15.12: In Case of Non-immune Hemolysis, Assess the Cause

Hemolysis due to freezing of pRBCs
Hemolysis due to inappropriate warming of pRBCs to higher temperature
Hemolysis due to transfusion of other IV fluid with same blood set

Box 15.13 Fix the Cause Due to Mechanical Damage of pRBC

Roller pumps used in cardiac surgery
Infusion under pressure through small-bore needle
Blood pumps

Perform ABO and Rh regrouping of "donor" blood from the blood bag and from the pilot tube separately, and repeat the crossmatch with both the samples with fresh sample of patient blood to find out any discrepancy (Box 15.14).

Box 15.14: In Case of ABO Mismatch, Ascertain the Cause Due to

Grouping error
Wrong blood in tube
Labelling error
Transfusion of wrong blood units

Examine the patient's serum for hemolysis.

Take second posttransfusion patient's blood sample 6 h after transfusion to determine serum bilirubin and hemoglobin level.

Repeat determining serum bilirubin level after 24 h.

Perform direct antiglobulin test with washed red cells of posttransfusion sample of the patient. A weak positive test is strongly indicative of incompatible blood transfusion (hemolytic reaction).

Table 15.9 Investigation summary for transfusion reaction

Investigations	Pretransfusion	Posttransfusion
Repeat ABO group of patient		
Repeat Rh group of patient		
Repeat ABO of the donor (pilot tube)		
Repeat Rh group of donor (pilot tube)		
Repeat crossmatch		
Repeat direct antiglobulin test		
Repeat antibody screen		
Hemoglobin of patient		
Test for hemoglobinuria		
Serum bilirubin level		
Platelet count		
Prothrombin time and INR		
Blood culture (sample from blood bag)		

Prepare a blood smear from the patient's blood following hemolytic reaction and stained with Leishman stain, and see the presence of microspherocytes or red cell fragments which is indicative of incompatibility.

Perform antibody screening of patient's serum for the presence of unusual antibody.

The diagnosis of suspected extravascular (delayed) hemolytic reaction is made by suspecting the possibility, repeating hematocrits for up to 3 weeks after post transfusion, checking bilirubin levels, and submitting new specimens to the blood bank to check the direct antiglobulin test (direct Coombs) and to find out antibody causing the reaction (Table 15.9).

For acute hemolytic transfusion reaction, check for visual hemolysis.

For delayed hemolytic transfusion reaction: Compare positive posttransfusion DAT to pretransfusion DAT.

Amnestic response: Appearance of alloantibody can occur within hours of exposure.

15.14.3 Acute Hemolytic Transfusion Reaction

In anesthetized patients, hypotension and evidence of disseminated intravascular coagulation (DIC) may be the first sign. This may be a fatal reaction.

15.14.3.1 Investigation

Clinically assess patients for common features of hemolysis occurring within 24 h of transfusion.

Check clerical records, such as ABO typing of patient and unit.

Repeat patient ABO grouping and antibody screen in both pre- and posttransfusion samples.

Perform direct antiglobulin test (DAT) and indirect antiglobulin test (IAT), renal function, and tests for hemolysis (e.g., serum haptoglobin).

Maintain blood pressure and renal output.

Induce diuresis with intravenous fluids and diuretics.

Further Reading

Bain BJ. Bloody easy: blood transfusions, blood alternatives and transfusion reactions: a guide to transfusion medicine. J Clin Pathol. 2005;58(6):672.

Benjamin RJ, McDonald CP, ISBT Transfusion Transmitted Infectious Disease Bacterial Workgroup. The international experience of bacterial screen testing of platelet components with an automated microbial detection system: a need for consensus testing and reporting guidelines. Transfus Med Rev. 2014;28(2):61–71.

Delaney M, Wendel S, Bercovitz RS, Cid J, Cohn C, Dunbar NM, Apelseth TO, Popovsky M, Stanworth SJ, Tinmouth A, Van De Watering L. Transfusion reactions: prevention, diagnosis, and treatment. Lancet. 2016;388(10061):2825–36.

Denise MH. Modern blood banking and transfusion practices, vol. 15. Philadelphia, PA: FA Davis Company; 2005. p. 208.

Doan CA. The transfusion problem. Physiol Rev. 1927;7(1):1–84.

Eder AF, Chambers LA. Noninfectious complications of blood transfusion. Arch Pathol Lab Med. 2007;131(5):708–18.

Eder AF, Dy BA, Kennedy JM, Notari EP IV, Strupp A, Wissel ME, Reddy R, Gibble J, Haimowitz MD, Newman BH, Chambers LA. The American Red Cross donor hemovigilance program: complications of blood donation reported in 2006. Transfusion. 2008;48(9):1809–19.

Hillyer CD, Josephson CD, Blajchman MA, Vostal JG, Epstein JS, Goodman JL. Bacterial contamination of blood components: risks, strategies, and regulation: joint ASH and AABB educational session in transfusion medicine. Hematology Am Soc Hematol Educ Program. 2003;2003(1):575–89.

Kim J, Na S. Transfusion-related acute lung injury; clinical perspectives. Korean J Anesthesiol. 2015;68(2):101.

Possible Risks of Blood Product Transfusions from American Cancer Society. Last Medical. Archived from https://www.cancer.org/treatment/treatments-and-side-effects/treatment-types/blood-transfusion-and-donation/how-blood-transfusions-are-done.html#:~:text=Possible%20risks%20of%20blood%20transfusions,now%20more%20common%20than%20infections.

Polizzotto MN, Wood EM, Ingham H, Keller AJ, Australian Red Cross Blood Service Donor and Product Safety Team. Reducing the risk of transfusion-transmissible viral infection through blood donor selection: the Australian experience 2000 through 2006. Transfusion. 2008;48(1):55–63.

Popovsky M, editor. Transfusion reactions. 4th ed. Bethesda: AABB Press; 2012.

Sorensen BS, Johnsen SP, Jorgensen J. Complications related to blood donation: a population-based study. Vox Sang. 2008;94(2):132–7.

Glossary

Additive solution Is a preservative solution specifically to retain the beneficial properties of plasma and cellular components of blood during storage.

Allogeneic donation Means collection of whole blood or blood components from an individual and intended for transfusion to another individual. It can also be used in pharma industry as a raw product for the manufacturing of different blood products for medicinal use.

Apheresis Is a procedure for obtaining different components by specialized machine processing of whole blood in which the residual components of the blood are returned to the donor during or at the end of the process.

Autologous donation Means collection of whole blood or its components from an individual and intended solely for subsequent transfusion to the same individual or other human application to the same individual.

Autologous transfusion Means a transfusion in which the donor and the recipient are the same person and in which pre-deposited blood or blood components are used.

Allogenic blood Means blood collected from a donor and processed either for transfusion or for further manufacturing of different blood components for further use.

Blood component Means different blood components such as packed red blood cells, fresh frozen plasma, platelets, buffy coat, cryoprecipitate, and others recovered from whole blood for therapeutic use.

Blood component release Means a protocol which enables a blood component to be released from a quarantine status by the use of hospital management systems and procedures to ensure that the finished product meets its release specification.

Blood product Means different blood components derived from whole blood or plasma.

Blood transfusion The technique of replacing blood and its components.

Buffy coat Is a blood component consisting of white blood cells and platelets.

Cryoprecipitate Is a plasma component prepared from fresh frozen plasma by freeze–thaw precipitation of proteins and subsequent concentration and resuspension of the precipitated proteins in a small volume of the plasma.

Cryopreservation Means prolongation of the storage life of blood components by freezing.

Deferral Means temporary or permanent contraindication of collection of blood or its components from an individual due to medical reasons.

Directed donation Is one in which potential recipient selects his own donors.

Distribution Means supply of blood and its components to other hospitals, blood banks, medical institutions and pharma companies for the manufacture of blood products other than issuing of blood or blood components for transfusion.

Granulocytes, apheresis Means a concentrated suspension of granulocytes obtained by apheresis.

Hemoglobin Is the oxygen transporting protein molecule that makes up 95% of a red cell.

P. S. Ajmani, *Immunohematology and Blood banking*, https://doi.org/10.1007/978-981-15-8435-0

Hemovigilance Is a set of organized surveillance procedures relating to serious adverse or unexpected reactions or events in donors or recipients, and the epidemiological followup of donors.

Hospital blood bank Means any medical establishment unit within a hospital which stores and distributes, and may perform different blood tests to assess the suitability of blood or its components, and supply of blood.

Imputability Means the likelihood that a serious adverse reaction in a recipient can be attributed to the blood or blood component transfused or that a serious adverse reaction in a donor can be attributed to the donation process.

Plasma Is the liquid portion of the blood from which cells have been removed.

Plasma, cryoprecipitate depleted for transfusion Means a plasma component prepared from a unit of plasma, fresh frozen. It comprises the residual portion after the cryoprecipitate has been removed.

Plasma derivatives Are concentrates of specific plasma proteins prepared by the process of fractionation of collected blood from pools of more than two donors of plasma. They are not prepared in blood bank but manufactured by pharma companies.

Plasma, fresh frozen Means the supernatant plasma separated from the whole blood, or plasma collected by apheresis, frozen and stored.

Platelets, apheresis Means a concentrated suspension of blood platelets obtained by apheresis.

Platelets, apheresis, leucocyte depleted Means a concentrated suspension of blood platelets, obtained by apheresis, and from which leucocytes are removed.

Platelets, recovered, pooled Means a concentrated suspension of blood platelets, obtained by processing of whole blood units and pooling the platelets from the units during or after separation.

Platelets, recovered, pooled, leucocyte-depleted Means a concentrated suspension of blood platelets, obtained by processing of whole blood units and pooling the platelets from the units during or after separation, and from which leucocytes are removed.

Platelets, recovered, single unit Means a concentrated suspension of blood platelets, obtained by processing of a single unit of whole blood.

Platelets, recovered, single unit, leucocyte-depleted Means a concentrated suspension of blood platelets, obtained by processing of a single whole blood unit from which leucocytes are removed.

Red cells (pRBCs) or RCC Means the concentrated red cells from a single whole blood donation minus plasma from the donated unit.

Red cells, apheresis Means the red cells from an apheresis red cell donation.

Red cells, buffy coat removed Means that the concentrated red cells from a single whole blood donation minus plasma, platelets, and leucocytes.

Red cells, buffy coat removed, in additive solution Means that the concentrated red cells from a single whole blood donation minus plasma, platelets, and leucocytes from the collected blood plus addition of nutrient or preservative solution.

Red cells in additive solution Means the red cell concentrate from a single whole blood donation, with a large proportion of the plasma from the donation removed. A nutrient or preservative solution is added.

Red cells, leucocyte-depleted Means the red cells from a single whole blood donation, with a large proportion of the plasma and leucocytes from the donation removed.

Red cells, leucocyte-depleted, in additive solution Means the red cells from a single whole blood donation, with a large proportion of the plasma and leucocytes from the donated unit have been removed. A nutrient or preservative solution is added.

Reporting year Means the period starting from 1st of April to 31st of March of year.

Serious adverse event Means any untoward occurrence associated with the collection, testing, processing, storage, and distribution of blood or blood components that might lead to death or life-threatening, disabling, or incapacitating conditions for patients or which results in, or prolongs, hospitalization or morbidity.

Serious adverse reaction Means an unintended response in a donor or in a patient associated with the collection or transfusion of blood or blood components that is fatal, life-threatening, disabling, or which results in, or prolongs, hospitalization or morbidity.

Statistical process control Means a method of quality control of a product or a process that relies on a system of analysis of an adequate sample size without the need to measure every product of the process.

Traceability Means the procedure to trace each individual unit of blood or blood component derived thereof from the donor to its final destination, whether this is a recipient, a manufacturer of medicinal products or disposal, and vice versa.

Validation Means the establishment of documented and objective evidence that the particular requirements for a specific intended use can be consistently fulfilled.

Washed Means a process of removing plasma or storage solution from whole blood by different methods.

Whole blood Means unseparated blood collected into an approved blood bag container containing an anticoagulant preservative solution.

Index

P. S. Ajmani, *Immunohematology and Blood banking*, https://doi.org/10.1007/978-981-15-8435-0

GPSR Compliance

The European Union's (EU) General Product Safety Regulation (GPSR) is a set of rules that requires consumer products to be safe and our obligations to ensure this.

If you have any concerns about our products, you can contact us on ProductSafety@springernature.com

In case Publisher is established outside the EU, the EU authorized representative is:

Springer Nature Customer Service Center GmbH
Europaplatz 3
69115 Heidelberg, Germany

Batch number: 10371059

Printed by Printforce, the Netherlands